Getting Together and Staying Together

Getting Together and Staying Together

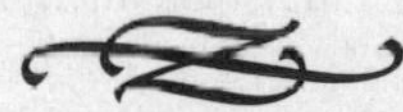

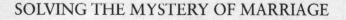

SOLVING THE MYSTERY OF MARRIAGE

WILLIAM GLASSER, M.D.,
AND CARLEEN GLASSER

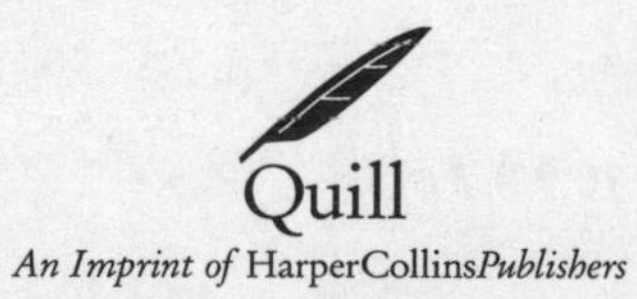

Quill
An Imprint of HarperCollins*Publishers*

TO CARLEEN'S PARENTS, CARL AND ISABEL, TOGETHER SINCE 1936

Previously published as *Staying Together.*

HarperCollins books may be purchased for educational, business, or sales promotional use. For information please write: Special Markets Department, HarperCollins Publishers Inc., 10 East 53rd Street, New York, NY 10022.

FIRST EDITION

Designed by Joy O'Meara

Library of Congress Cataloging-in-Publication Data

Glasser, William, 1925–
Getting together and staying together : solving the mystery of marriage / William Glasser and Carleen Glasser—1st ed.
p. cm.
Earlier ed. published in 1995 under title: Staying together.
ISBN 0-06-095633-X
1. Marriage. 2. Man-woman relationships. 3. Control theory.
I. Glasser, Carleen. II. Glasser, William. Staying together. III. Title.
HQ734. G546 2000
306.81—dc21 00-026206

01 02 03 04 ❖/RRD 10 9 8 7 6 5 4 3

Contents

How This Book Came to Be

Late in 1992, Naomi, my wife of forty-six years, died of cancer after a brief illness. We had a good marriage and were especially close for the six months that she was ill. Before she died, we talked honestly about the future and how I would conduct my life with regard to our children, grandchildren, assets, and work, and I have followed through on what I promised. We also discussed my personal life. Knowing me so well, she announced that I would need a new companion and said, "I hope you find the right one." I didn't anticipate that the loneliness would be so acute, but she was right. After all those years of marriage, I was an unhappy bachelor.

There are a lot of advantages to looking for love at an age when many of love's usual problems—money, children, not enough free time—are behind you. Still, finding someone was not easy. I met several fine women, but the right one eluded me. Then I got lucky. I found my current wife, Carleen. From this wonderful relationship, we've both learned a lot. To share that knowledge, with Carleen's help, I wrote the 1995 book, *Staying Together*.

In the year 2000, Carleen and I will have been married for five years and together for almost seven. During that time, we have barely had a cross word, and our marriage is stronger than ever. What we have accomplished is not luck. From the beginning, we decided to base our relationship on what I then called control theory, a theory that we had both used and taught for years.

We wrote this book, a new edition of *Staying Together*, because we have learned a lot about marriage by being married. From what we've learned, we have expanded and clarified the original control theory and given it a much more accurate name: *choice theory*. Not surprisingly, choice theory grew out of the long-held belief that all of our behavior is chosen. Further, the underlying motivation for everything we choose to do is genetic. Therefore, driven by our genes, what we do with our lives is not random: It is purposeful. And it is always our best effort at the time we choose it.

In this book, we explain what we have learned from putting choice theory to work in every aspect of our relationship and how our compatible connection has become a successful marriage. There is every reason to believe that what we've done can be done by any reasonably compatible couple who loved each other when they got married. What destroys marriages is neither incompatibility nor lack of love. It is the destructive behavior each partner adopts soon after marriage. Once they choose these behaviors, it is inevitable they will continue, and over time, both partners will become miserable.

The subtitle of this book is *Solving the Mystery of Marriage* because, for the vast majority of people, what begins to reduce their affection for each other after marriage is a total mystery. Couples whose marriages started out full of love, couples who couldn't get enough of each other in the beginning, see that early closeness begin to slip away, and they haven't the slightest idea of what's going wrong. The warm feeling for each other may return in brief spurts, and other parts of their marriage, such as closeness to their family and friends, may remain satisfying, but their personal relationship either continues to deteriorate or stabilizes at a level well below their initial expectations.

As the years go by, many divorce, but even more stay together trapped in a joyless tedium often made tolerable only by escaping with the help of alcohol, food, drugs, or affairs. If you are in or approaching this situation, don't despair. Read on, and you will learn how you can regain the closeness you once had—if you are willing to make the effort. But we have to warn you: This will take some effort. You may have to start living your life differently from the way you have lived it since birth. We also want to say that the characters in this book are fictional, but they are based on real people.

My Marriage Is a Mystery

A while back we received the following e-mail:

> *To: wginst@earthlink.net*
> *From: Cherylm@mail.anywhere.com*
> *Subject: query on marriage*
>
> I have sent this query to the websites of several well-known psychologists and psychiatrists, but to tell you the truth, I'm not even sure I want an answer. I'm even worried that what you may tell me will make me feel worse than I feel now. The other possibility is that there isn't an answer; there certainly doesn't seem to be one. I won't be surprised if you tell me that the marriage I have is the way marriage is and I should just accept it.
>
> To begin, I guess the best way to put it is, that for

me, marriage is a mystery. It became a mystery a few years after we married, and in the twenty-plus years I've been married to Larry, my husband, it remains a mystery. Larry doesn't know I'm writing this letter, but as far as I can see, it's as much a mystery to him as it is to me. On the surface, we have a good marriage. We don't fight or argue much and, I guess compared to their marriages, my friends tell me I have one of the best marriages in our circle. But it's not good enough for me.

My problem is that there's no spark in our relationship. To put it in two words: It's dull. There's nothing to look forward to. It just goes along month after month, the ups never high, the lows rarely low. Our marriage reminds me of the heart monitor on *ER* when the patient dies, flat, no more beeps. It's not that we don't do things or see people we enjoy. But the enjoyment is more as individuals than as a couple. For example, with our friends he's with the men and I'm with the women. What we don't seem to be able to do anymore is enjoy each other. When we're together by ourselves, there's no real substance to our relationship.

More and more, I think about the beginning, about how much in love we were. How every moment we could spend together was so precious. How just being with each other seemed to be all we needed. It's not that I have any hope we could ever recapture those initial feelings, but this is too far in the other direction. As I look over what I've just written, it sounds stupid. Why would you be interested in the complaints of a disgruntled forty-two-year-old woman? I feel stupid for even bothering you.

Anyway, here's the conclusion I've come to after wracking my brain for a year. And mind you, all I can really speak for are wives. I don't think I know that much about how my husband really feels or what he thinks about, and neither do the women I've discussed this with. If we had that kind of communication in the first place, we'd have much better marriages. When I ask them, most women say, "I'm happily married." And I say it, too. But what we are talking about is the whole picture: friends, family, children, grandchildren, and even the people we work with. What we don't talk about is happiness with our husbands.

So I'm not saying it's all bad. We have the status of being married, which is still important to most women, and my guess is to most men. It's certainly important to me. Marriage gives us more money, help with our children, and a man we can trust in a crisis, much more than we would have if we weren't married. And in so many marriages in our circle, our husbands are like Larry, good men whom we loved when we married them and for whom we still have some affection if no longer any passion.

I would also say that most women don't even want to face what I've written here. As I said, I'm almost afraid to send this to you: I dread that you'll tell me that what I have is as good as it's going to get. Tone down your expectations; the part of your life that you long for is over. You've got a good husband, make the best of it, you could be a lot worse off than you are.

Well, I've decided not to settle for what I have. I'm not going to settle for the marriage I have without trying to find out more than I know now. I'm sick of this being such a mystery—there must be things I can do. I'm also willing to put some effort into any suggestion you may give me that makes sense. Please, if you have anything to tell me, I'd like to hear from you.

Cheryl M.

Since Carleen and I had just completed the first six chapters of this book, Cheryl's letter couldn't have been more timely. We quickly e-mailed our response.

We offered to send Cheryl the chapters but warned her that just reading them wouldn't solve her problems. Repairing a relationship isn't a simple "Do this" or "Don't do that" situation. It requires work *and change,* and it requires the willing participation of both partners.

We urged Cheryl to show Larry her e-mail and ours, and to get back to us if Larry was onboard. We also thanked her for giving us the subtitle to our book: *Solving the Mystery of Marriage.*

2

Larry's Dilemma

The day after we e-mailed our answer to Cheryl, I got a call from her husband, Larry. As soon as she got our reply, Cheryl had shared both e-mails with him. They had a long talk, and after overcoming some doubts and a little denial, they agreed they'd both really like to have a better marriage. They decided they were willing to work at it together. He then told me the reason for his call. He wanted to talk with me before I sent the manuscript so I'd have a better idea of what he thought was wrong with their marriage.

Since Carleen and I live and work in our home in West Los Angeles, Larry asked if I would be willing to come south, closer to where he worked in Orange County. He wanted to meet with me professionally so that what we talked about could be kept confidential. He didn't care if I shared it with Carleen, but he didn't want Cheryl to find out what he told me. She had shared our letter with him, so I could see no reason not to listen to what he had to say. I agreed to meet him the next day for lunch.

When I got to the restaurant, he was already sitting at a table. The restaurant was not crowded, so there would be no problem with privacy. He was a nice-looking man, trim and tanned, who smiled as if he was glad to see me. We introduced ourselves, exchanged a little small talk for a moment while the waiter got us some water, and then went to the buffet to get our lunch. When we got back to the table he began to eat and talk.

Larry was a professor at a large state college not far from where he lived. He'd been at the college for almost his whole married life. He enjoyed teaching and was respected in his field. His wife was the director of a nursery school near where they lived. It was pretty much as she'd described in her letter: no major problems with health, money; their two children were away at college and getting along well. But he agreed with her that there was not much companionship and very little sex. By the time we finished lunch, I had learned a lot about Larry and his life with Cheryl but, as far as I could see, nothing that needed to be kept secret from anyone. He then ordered coffee, and I waited for him to tell me why he had wanted so much to see me.

He hesitated a moment and then said, "You know, Doctor, I'm glad my wife wrote you, and I'm looking forward to reading your manuscript. We'll read it together. But I have to tell you, I have some doubts that a book could help our marriage. I'd like to tell you why, if it's okay with you."

I nodded for him to go ahead.

"When she wrote you that we were in love in the beginning, she told the truth. We were. And I think she still loves me, whatever that means after twenty years of the kind of marriage we've had. And for what it's worth, I still love her. But maybe what I'm saying is that I still love the woman she was when we got married. And, like she still has hopes about me, I haven't given up hope she could be that woman again. Once in a while we have a few days of closeness, but it never lasts. It may be my fault that it doesn't last, but it's the way she is that makes it so hard for me. As soon as we have a little closeness, she wrecks it for me. To be honest, I don't think she has any idea what she does that turns me off so much. Do you have any idea what I'm trying to tell you?"

"I really don't. Go ahead, tell me what you came to tell me."

"I'm trying. The problem is, now that I'm here, it's real hard to explain what bothers me without sounding like a jerk. I'm worried that I'll come across as shallow and intolerant, and I don't really think I am."

"I can't predict how you'll come across to me; you'll have to take a chance on that. But I'm curious. I'd like to hear what you're having so much trouble saying. Besides, I don't look at people who come to see me as shallow or as deep. I look at them as people struggling to get as much as they can out of their lives. And often, in the process doing things that hurt the people they care for. Maybe hurting themselves, too. It's pain that brings people to see me. I think it's pain that brought you here."

"It *is* pain. I didn't notice it so much years ago when it started, but now it's there almost all the time. It's not acute or something I can't stand, just kind of a dull, gnawing ache, something that feels as if it's never going to go away.

What I haven't been able to come to terms with is that Cheryl's a complainer. Not so much to other people, but to me, about everything. She doesn't always complain *about* me, but I can't help but think that it's directed at me, anyway. Doctor, the complaints are constant; nothing is ever the way it should be."

"Have you told her it bothers you?"

"I have, but she just says it's the way she is, that I shouldn't pay attention to it, but I do, I can't help it. Whenever she complains, I can't help thinking I have to fix it or take care of it. She tells me I don't, but I get desperate to stop her complaints, so I keep trying to fix what I can. It's a losing battle, like spitting in the ocean. She keeps telling me to stop trying to fix things. She admits she doesn't want solutions, she just wants me to listen to her. But even that isn't easy. Look, we go out for dinner in a neighborhood restaurant. On the way, the traffic's too heavy, the parking's terrible, the table's not ready or it's too close to the kitchen or it's too noisy. The food is good but it's late and it's not hot. And the service is so slow we're going to miss the movie she wanted so much to see. I don't even think she notices it, but there's something wrong with everything and everyone, and I have to hear about it all."

"Do you think you're blowing it out of proportion?"

"Maybe. Maybe I am exaggerating, but not that much. Even when she isn't complaining, it doesn't seem to help because I expect it and get tense waiting for what I know is going to happen. I find myself walking on eggs, trying to fix things before they happen, trying to take responsibility for the whole imperfect world that she can't abide. And getting frustrated because I can't. She even complains that I go off to work too happy in the morning, and she's right, I do. I've also gotten to the point where I never complain about anything because when I do she one-ups me, what happened to her was so much worse than what happened to me."

"What happens if you start out by saying it's our lucky day, everything is fine?"

"Like I said, I used to try, but I've given up. She gets angry and calls me a wimp. She says if it weren't for her, people would walk all over me."

"Have you thought about divorce?"

"Of course I've thought about divorce. But I'm not painting the whole picture. She does a lot more than complain. She takes care of me. She tells me I need care and she gives it to me. She doesn't seem to resent taking care of me at all. She almost never complains about that. But she also takes care of everyone in the family, really does a lot for them and then complains to me about all she has to do. But still she likes to take care of people. She's happy when she does, even with all the complaints. She also runs a perfect home. She's a great cook. She operates a top-notch nursery school, never complains about the kids and never fails to complain about their parents. If I'm sick or need anything, she's there and she complains that I don't need her enough. And she's loyal. She doesn't have much interest in what I do, but she supports my job and complains that people don't appreciate me enough. I'm afraid to tell her about any of my troubles at work because it'll set her off. But, Doctor, I can't leave her. She's a good person who lives in a lousy world. And if she could be in charge, I really think it'd be a better world, but she'll never be in charge. Besides, I love her. We've been together for so many years, I just can't picture my life without her. As much as she complains, she's more on my side than anyone else is. She's not the kind of person you'd want to lose."

"I guess it may have helped you to tell me all you've just told me, but I get the feeling that you still haven't told me what you really came here for."

"No, I haven't. I haven't told anyone. I can't. It's how I deal with her, how I put up with all her complaining. I want to stop doing it. I'm hoping just as much as she is that what you've written will help us to get along better. I want to tell you this so you know she's not the only one at fault in our marriage. I'm more at fault than she is. I lead a double life. It's what keeps me going. I rationalize what I do by telling myself that once in a while I deserve to get away from all her complaints, that it's her fault I do what I'm doing. But of course it isn't. I do it because I want to do it. And I have no intention of doing anything more than I'm doing. I never plan to leave her or even give her a hard time. I treat her well, but she's right when she says there's no real close feeling between us. Or maybe it's me who doesn't feel close to her. I'm not blaming her, Doctor, but if she'd stop complaining, things between us would be a lot better."

I just kept looking at him.

"I don't need closeness with her because I get it from other women. I have long-term affairs where I get to know the women very well. But again, what I have with them is superficial. They're not part of my life and I'm really not part of theirs. They supplement Cheryl, but they don't replace her. They don't and they never will."

"Where do you find these women?"

"There are plenty at the college where I work. They're just like me. Mostly they're married and have no intention of leaving their husbands or families, but they lack intimacy in their marriages, too. Like me, they're well aware of what they need and what I can give. We tread a narrow line; we accept that to need or want more'll destroy what we have. They need their husbands and families, really, their marriages, as much as I need mine. If they're divorced, they need me until they find someone permanent. It's like I've detached sex and closeness from my marriage. What I'm hoping is that you have something to offer that will help me to get back into my marriage what I've separated out of it. The closeness, you know what I mean? Do you understand what I'm trying to tell you?"

"They settle for what you give them? They don't want more?"

"I'm sure many women who have affairs want more, but I've gotten pretty good at recognizing the kind of person I want, and I put my cards on the table first. In the ten years I've led this life, I've made very few mistakes and none so severe that it's caused me or the woman any real problems."

"They never tell their husbands or anyone else?"

"Doctor, when it comes to illicit sex and love, I've found that women are realists. They keep their mouths shut. It's the men who are the romantics, who fall in love and screw everything up. And I'm not in a hurry. If it takes some time to find someone, it's fine with me. I'm not looking for one-night stands. It's closeness and a kind of personal loyalty to what we have that I'm looking for as much as the sex. I'm very careful. And the women I've been with are equally careful. But still, I'd like to stop. I think I'm ready to try to stop. Maybe even more than Cheryl, I'm hoping what you and your wife have written will help me to stop. But like Cheryl said in her letter, there *is* a mystery to marriage. Why can't men and women find in their mates what they seem to find in affairs? My present woman and I talk about it and, like me, she says she was in love when she got married and to some extent she still is. Like me, she'd like to feel with her husband what she feels with me. I know her husband; he's not an ogre. What goes wrong? And here's the most mysterious part of all. Some of the women have been married before and it happened to them with the second and third husband just like with the first. Why can't people like me and the women I meet find what we find with each other in our marriages? What is it about marriage that seems to render this so difficult? Or is it impossible?"

"All I can tell you, Larry, is that what you've just asked me and what Cheryl asked in her letter are what Carleen and I are trying to answer in our book. We think there *is* an answer. We'd like you both to read the book and, if it makes sense, talk about it. It'll take some real effort, but try to make it a part of your marriage. Then send us a letter telling us what you think you've learned. You've been married twenty years, you don't want a divorce, there's no reason for you to hurry, you have plenty of time. This is a mystery that's not going to be solved quickly. And please be assured that what you've just told me will be kept completely confidential."

3

Getting Rid of External Control Psychology, the Marriage Killer

The marital relationship itself is a major source of unhappiness. There is no other relationship that attempts to lock together for life two adults who may know very little about each other apart from the fact that they are sexually attracted. In fact, one of the results of so many couples living together before marriage is that at the end of several years one or both decides he or she doesn't want to get married. What they are saying is, I don't want to lock myself in a relationship with you. But many of these couples do fall in love and marry, and still they experience what Cheryl wrote to me about. So even living together does not prepare a couple for the bound-together relationship that is marriage.

Marriage asks more of its partners than does any other relationship. At the same time, it prepares its partners less for what could go wrong. What couples need to know before marriage, what Carleen and I knew before we married, is nowhere near common knowledge. Marriage is entered into by people who wouldn't think of entering into a business partnership without laying out in detail, usually in writing, how to handle problems that may arise. It is this kind of preparation for being married that this book is all about.

When Cheryl and Larry got married, they were in love, they already were or soon would be sexually active, and they may have felt better than they had ever felt in their lives. Neither could conceive that in less than ten years they would find themselves mired in a joyless personal relationship with no idea of what to do to revive it. They stayed together because of all the other good parts of marriage and because they were unwilling to chance the even greater pain of separation or divorce.

There is nothing exceptional about Cheryl and Larry's marital experience. A good marriage is the most difficult of all affiliations to maintain. A little over half of all who marry are able to stay married for life. And of those who do, very few achieve the storybook ending of living happily ever after. A long-term happy marriage is the least successful of all our relationships.

But like Larry and Cheryl, who are asking us for help, countless unhappy couples spend both time and money trying to find out how to revive their failing marriage. They seek help ranging from "Dear Abby" to therapy, but much of this help is ineffective, usually because they are waiting for the experts to tell them how to straighten out their partners. Few of the experts teach them what we explain in this book: No matter what shape their relationship is in, they can change only themselves.

The reason that people like Cheryl and Larry find marriage so unrewarding is that when they have difficulty getting along with each other, they practice what I call *external control psychology.* And they are far from alone in this practice. External control is practiced by 99.99 percent of the people in the world when they have trouble getting along with someone else. It is hardly exclusive to marriage, but of all the harm it does, it saves its most severe for marriage.

External control has this as its major premise: *If we are unhappy, we are not responsible for the way we feel. It's always other people, events we can't control, or something structurally or chemically wrong with our brain that is the cause of our pain. It is never what we choose to do that is the cause of our misery.* Employing external control, unhappily married people keep thinking: *It's not me, it's my partner who's the cause of my misery. And it's my obligation to do everything I can to change the way my partner behaves toward me up to and including killing him or her.*

To satisfy this "obligation," we very often choose a stereotypical group of behaviors that I call **the Seven Deadly Habits** of external control psychology. I call them stereotypical because almost all of us choose them over and over without giving much thought to how much misery they cause us and others. These are (1) *criticizing,* (2) *blaming,* (3) *complaining,* (4) *nagging,* (5) *threatening,* (6) *punishing,* and (7) *bribing or rewarding to control.* These habits are deadly because, given enough time, their persistent use kills any marriage. We discuss these habits further in Chapter 5.

The couple may not divorce, but they find themselves in the same situation as Cheryl and Larry, or worse. Try going a day without using any of the habits; this is almost impossible to do. It's so hard because in the situations in which you use them, as Larry complained to me about Cheryl, it is almost impossible to consider doing anything else.

Therefore, as we seek help from friends or even professionals, almost all of whom follow external control themselves, we gain support for what we already believe: *We are involved with the wrong mate, or if we decide to stay, he or she must change if we are to be happy*. And since it's the other person's fault, not ours, we don't try to change our own behavior. So our unhappiness continues and usually increases. To make the changes needed for a better marriage, we must learn a lot more about ourselves and about the psychology we use than we know now.

What my wife and I offer is a new psychology, *choice theory,* that you can begin to use immediately—not only in your marriage but in every aspect of your life—to replace the universally destructive *external control* that now dominates your behavior. This new psychology is called *choice theory* because it teaches that we choose all we do or feel, including our misery. So if we want to feel better, we must change the way we choose to live our lives. In most instances, this means we must take a careful look at what we do when we have difficulty getting along with other people.

For example, if I were Larry, I would say to myself, *I must look carefully at everything I do in my personal relationship with Cheryl and make sure that I am not using external control. If I can do this, I will avoid doing anything that will move us farther apart than we are now. In fact, I must try to do everything I can to bring us closer together, and to do that I must begin to use choice theory in all I say or do with her.* If I were Cheryl, I would do exactly the same thing with Larry. If only one partner does this, it may help a little, but the real power is in doing it together.

Excluding some very good family relationships, the only other close adult relationships we have besides marriage are with our long-term friends. What is extremely interesting about these two affiliations is that marriage is the least successful adult relationship, whereas long-term friendships are by far the most successful. The reason for this difference is clear: External control is more widely used in marriage than in any other relationship. In contrast, external control is almost never used in a long-term friendship.

In fact, long-term friendships are the only human relationships where, without knowing that we are doing it, we use choice theory from the start. And as long as we continue to use it, our friendships remain strong. This is the reason that long-term friendships are the longest and strongest of all human relationships.

I've often asked unhappily married couples who've come for help, "Why don't you treat your friends the way you treat each other?" They almost always answer, "If I treated my friends that way, I'd lose them." Pointing this out to a couple who want a happier marriage can be a great help toward getting them to think seriously about replacing external control with choice theory. But the difficulty is that there is almost no awareness of how harmful external control is anywhere in our society. And, equally, there is little awareness anywhere of what choice theory is or how it can be used to replace external control.

If we take a detailed look at why friendship is more successful than marriage, it is easy to see that the destructive hand of external control is associated with every difference between these two relationships. The first difference is obvious. Unlike friendship, marriage is legally, morally, and often religiously binding. Its whole foundation is built on external control, on coercive forces designed to keep the marriage intact. But there is little or no happiness in control as epitomized in: *What God hath joined together let no man put asunder no matter how miserable this relationship turns out to be.*

Carleen and I are against neither marriage nor divorce. What we are against is the external control that destroys marriage and leads to divorce. Totally unlike marriage, a long-term friendship is, at most, only morally binding; there is no sworn commitment, no attempt to force a friend to do anything he or she doesn't want to do. For success, friendship depends only on both parties agreeing to honor it. When they stop, it is over. There is never any attempt at control. And in the era of no-fault divorce it is clear that any attempts to force people to stay married cause more problems than they solve.

A second difference is that marriage obligates physical closeness. Married people "should" live together or, if apart, stay in close touch. Long-term friends neither need to live close nor stay in constant touch with each other to maintain the friendship.

A third difference is that unlike a failing friendship, marriage is filled with tangible penalties that kick in as soon as it fails. Among these are spousal support, child support, visitation rights, religious or social ostracism, alienation of family members, and loss of property. But couples who know they will suffer all the above penalties still break up almost always because they can't accept the degree of control that marriage imposes. We are not against any of these legal protections. What we are for is more successful marriages.

Finally, psychological problems that are mostly caused by controlling or being controlled, such as what are usually thought of as mental illness, addictions such as alcoholism, and violence such as spousal and child abuse, are common to failing and failed marriages. Such problems are totally foreign to long-term friendships. In fact, good long-term friends are more helpful in preventing mental and behavioral problems than any other person except loving family members.

Therefore, external control is the destroyer of marriages. As long as we practice it, there is little chance we will have any more marital success than we have now. If Larry and Cheryl can learn enough choice theory to put it to work in their marriage, they have a good chance of reviving what seemed to them, when they wrote to us, an almost hopeless situation. But even more, we believe that if Cheryl and Larry had known before they got married what we will now attempt to teach them, they would not have found themselves in the situation they are in. At this point, to give you a picture of how we used choice theory from the beginning of our relationship, I'll turn the story over to Carleen.

4

Carleen's Story

I am no stranger to marital unhappiness. More years than I care to admit were wasted in a loveless union with a partner I did not relate to and who didn't seem to relate to me. A recurrent question I asked myself over all those years was, What do I want that I'm not getting? I thought I was getting what I wanted when I married, but I was totally mistaken. Like many people, I had no idea what I wanted in a relationship before I got married, so it stands to reason that I married the wrong person. Often, I asked myself what I was doing to contribute to my marriage problems. But it remained a complete mystery to me. My head was full of thoughts like, If only he would change, I would be so much happier.

Then, in 1983, I read *Reality Therapy* by William Glasser. At that moment I began an exciting journey that would change the course of my life forever. By 1989, I had read every book Dr. Glasser had ever written and had completed all the training offered through his institute. I was now a basic week instructor in his institute, and in 1990 I wrote a book to teach his ideas to elementary-school children.

That same year, the institute's annual convention was held in my hometown, Cincinnati. As an instructor, I was actively involved in planning the convention with my friends Sandie and Bob Wubbolding. Bob had been my counseling professor at Xavier University in 1983 and was responsible for introducing me to *Reality Therapy* while I was his student and he was training me through the certification process over the next few years.

During the convention planning in Cincinnati, I got to know Naomi Glasser, and we became quite friendly. It was her job to coordinate the conventions in the various cities each year. She was good at it, and I admired and respected her a lot. Two and a half years later she died of cancer. Her loss was met throughout the organization with disbelief and great sadness. I had hardly gotten to know her, and she was gone. I can remember thinking at the time about what Dr. Glasser would do now without her.

The following year, I found myself engulfed in the pain and turmoil of a marriage that was breaking up, with all the tears and anger that accompanies it. Even though I had known for a few years that divorce was inevitable, I was unprepared for it when it happened. All along I'd realized what was missing in my life: happiness. I had financial success and professional fulfillment, but I was unhappy.

I recall saying something prophetic the summer before my divorce. One of my colleagues at the institute and I were talking over dinner one evening about relationships and how what we teach applies to everything we do.

Suddenly I turned to her and said, "You know what, Kathy, I wish I could be in a relationship with a man who understands what we teach."

Talk about a self-fulfilling prophecy! News of my divorce reached Dr. Glasser through the institute's grapevine. About a week later I received a lovely letter from Dr. Glasser telling me he'd heard about my divorce and asking me if I'd be interested in seeing him. Needless to say, I was astonished and delighted. The person I most admired in the whole world was saying the feeling was mutual. Of course I said yes, and as the saying goes, that was the beginning of the rest of my life. My personal past became a blur, except for my marvelous son and daughter, whom I adore, and my incredible parents and sister, without whose love my life would be empty.

By the end of our first date, I actually began to feel comfortable enough to call Dr. Glasser by his first name. Soon this wonderful man became the love of my life. I've never been this focused, this completely and passionately consumed by love for a man. Thoughts of Bill come first every waking hour of every day. It's simply a joy to be with him. He's funny. I laugh a lot. He's a genius. I think a lot—we think together. I think because he thinks. He says I'm brilliant. I love it. And on days when I don't see it, he holds a mirror up to me so I can.

In the beginning, I used to whine occasionally when I talked to him, kind of a whimpering babble of emotional insecurities. Bill calls it my squeaking period. Now I speak up with confidence and conviction, and he applauds. He defends me against my own self-criticism. He says, "Carleen, you can always get away from others when they criticize you, but you can never get away from yourself."

He's taught me to let the painful past go and not blame anyone, including myself. You learn most from your successes in life, not from your failures. Commiserating over past failure is a waste of precious time that could be used to create a more satisfying present. Bill has taught me how to be happy. I watch him using choice theory behaviors every day, and I'm learning how. It keeps us close; we're on the same wavelength.

When we got married in 1995, I was happy about moving to Los Angeles, but I was also leaving everything—friends and family, my hometown where I'd lived all my life. We were going to live in Bill's house, the one he and Naomi had lived in for more than forty years. His children had grown up there. I would have preferred to find another house—my house—to make a fresh start with Bill. But he wanted more than anything else to stay in his house.

This, our first conflict, was a real challenge to our decision to use choice theory in our marriage. He resisted any suggestions to change anything in the house. I recognized that for him, this house and everything in it was very much a part of his cherished past and present world. My love for him and my understanding of the concept of external control helped me deal with this conflict of wants. I knew it would hurt the wonderful relationship we had begun if I tried to force him to leave his house. I moved in, and little by little I pointed out to Bill what I imagined would help me feel more a part of his world. This sharing proved to be very helpful. We came to the conclusion that redecorating the house would match my picture of the home I wanted to create for us. He gave me the checkbook and said I should write all the checks (he hates writing big checks!). He said if I was happy, he'd be getting what he wanted.

We negotiated a solution to that conflict that worked out well for both of us. He got to stay where he wanted to live, and I got to create a beautiful new space for a fresh start. He loved the new look, and I enjoyed the satisfaction of knowing that he had something he wanted very much—including an ecstatic wife. All other decisions that we make in our marriage are made together by telling each other what we want and what we are willing to do that will help solve any problem or conflict of ideas. It works. Understanding choice theory has demystified marriage for me, and I have truly found what I've always wanted in a relationship: being successful at it and knowing why.

5

The Basic Needs: How They Relate to Marital Happiness

It is safe to say that all living organisms, from viruses to us, behave from birth to death. And the primary motivation for every bit of this huge variety of behavior is programmed into the organism's genes. The difference between us and animals, who are genetically similar to us and have needs recognizably similar to ours, is that we have no genetic programs that tell us how to behave to satisfy our needs. Even in higher animals like chimpanzees, a great many behaviors are programmed into their genes, and they don't behave much beyond where their genes take them. For all the jokes about chimpanzees with typewriters, they will never write *War and Peace*.

With the possible exception of angering, we have no built-in behaviors. We have to learn everything we do, and the motivation for this learning is our pleasurable and painful feelings. The better we do it, the better we feel, and this doing better and feeling better is the driving force behind all human progress. We may argue about what progress is—I'm sure somebody felt good when the pyramids were built—but that argument will never be won. Animals feel good if they can find sex, food, and safety. But for them, progress ends there. For us, driven by the hope of feeling better, it never ends. If I were asked what distinguishes us from all other life on earth, I would answer, progress.

For example, like all other animals, we are genetically programmed to engage in sex. But animals do not have to learn how to do it. While I'm sure it feels good when they do it, they, unlike us, are not programmed to try to do it better or more often. So the sex they engage in does not vary that much during their lives. But we have no such genetic stops. We engage in sex more than any other creature, we attempt to do it better and more often, and we are always hoping it will feel better than the last time we did it. A huge amount of human activity is devoted to thinking about sex and doing it. People spend more money on pornographic films than on all the other films produced, including blockbusters like *Titanic*.

All progress is the result of some people—usually only a few, often only one—attempting to feel better, or trying to avoid feeling bad, as they attempt to satisfy what I believe are five basic human needs built into our genes. These needs, in the order we will explain them in this book, are survival, love and belonging, power, freedom, and fun. While this simple genetic system has worked remarkably well for many human beings in that they feel happy, healthy, and satisfied—or if they don't, they aspire to feel happy, healthy, and satisfied—it has not worked well for marriage.

In the United States right now, fewer than half the people who are married feel happy, healthy, and satisfied. Marriage is an institution designed to help men and women satisfy their basic needs, but it does not work that way. There is no evidence anywhere that any significant group of married people in this country are getting along any better now than they did a hundred years ago. But we believe that if more married people understood that they are driven by the five basic needs and, using choice theory, made an effort in their marriage from the start to satisfy them, we could begin to make some significant progress in improving marriage.

For example, driven by one of our basic needs, *love and belonging,* we become more and more aware of the social consequences of our behavior. Nowhere is this awareness more acute than when we marry. Both Cheryl and Larry are well aware that when they criticize, blame, or complain about each other, they feel bad. But they have continued to do it for almost twenty years and, in that time, have squandered the love they used to have.

What they are not aware of is that the external control they both continue to use is the problem. The external control they have used since shortly after they married has not only made it hard for them to satisfy their need for love and belonging, it also has made it hard for them to satisfy their other needs. What we'll do now is explain the needs, starting with survival, obviously a need that all living creatures share.

Survival: The Marital Problems Associated with Money

In modern America, most people are assured of survival if they make any effort at all. Few people die of starvation or because they don't have a home. But as I explain in detail in a later chapter, people have different amounts of the need for survival programmed into their genes. Actually, this difference follows a normal distribution, as do all things in nature. Commonly, this difference shows itself in one being much more conservative than the other, and this trait is most often expressed by being more careful about money. As a rule, poverty is an obstacle to all happiness, and marriage is no exception to that rule. The old Joe E. Lewis quote, *I've been rich and I've been poor, and believe me, rich is better,* gets the most laughs from married people.

In many marriages the most common symptom of differences in the need to survive is fighting about money. And once a married couple begins to fight seriously about anything, their chance for a happy marriage diminishes. You may have noticed that when my wife wanted to redecorate our house, I solved my frugality problem by not even looking at the checks. It seems silly, but it worked. I am an older, raised-in-the-Great-Depression kind of person and more concerned about money than I should be. She isn't, but we solved the problem. What really helped is that we had a choice-theory mechanism for working out our differences that most people don't have. I explain that later in this chapter.

Love and Belonging: The Genetic Core of a Happy Marriage

A good marriage is probably the best vehicle to satisfy our need for love and belonging over the long haul. But being the best vehicle still doesn't make it easy to access because, unlike survival, we need another person to do it with. And as I have already begun to explain, we have no control over other people's behavior. You can't make another person love you, and any effort to force your love on someone else rarely works. It also may come as a surprise to many people who feel that they are in love that loving someone else does not necessarily persuade that person to love you.

Women, probably based on their role as mothers, seem to be endowed with a stronger need to love and belong than men. In practice this means they want to give more, but there may not be much difference in how much they want to receive. Based on this genetic difference, women often find themselves married to men who don't give them as much love as they want. In this situation, both partners are frustrated. She, because he doesn't give her enough; he, because his lesser need makes it difficult for him to understand why she both gives and wants so much.

But because the man has a lesser need does not prevent him from learning to give more. My genes may have made me naturally frugal, but I was able to learn to be more liberal with my money. The genes give us a level of need intensity, but they do not restrict us from overriding that level and feeling better (or worse) when we do. The way I see it, if a woman wants more than the man is genetically inclined to give, she has two choices: She can act on her frustration and become even more demanding (and less lovable) or, in a variety of ways, she can teach him to experience the joy of giving her more.

In the beginning of a marriage, many partners, especially women, are fooled by sex into believing that the men love them more than they actually do. This is because for women, unlike for men, sex is more genetically tied to their need for love than to their need to survive. A man with a strong survival need wants a lot of sex and, in the beginning, acts loving to get it.

But as the marriage continues, the woman usually sees through this act and realizes that the man loves sex as much or more than he loves her, and she becomes less interested in this hormonal, less loving act. As she loses interest, the man becomes more frustrated and demands more sex, which turns her off further, and the marriage deteriorates. To demand anything in marriage is a turnoff, and sex is no exception. We address this problem in the next chapter.

There is another very common problem with differences in the need for love. A woman with a very strong need for love recognizes that her partner needs less love, and she is more attracted, even challenged, by this difference. Driven by her strong need for love, she believes she will be able to love him so much that her love will bring out a latent need she is sure is there. Sometimes she succeeds, literally teaches him to love more. But in most cases, if she is too insistent and tries too hard, she fails. Teaching a man to love more than he feels naturally is a slow, careful process. It can't be hurried.

There are many individual variations of the need for love and belonging that tend to make marriage a mystery. Many women and men are very loving toward children yet seem unable to love an adult with the same intensity. This may be because children, especially small children, need so much attention and care, which is very satisfying to give, and parents do not expect to get very much in return from a small child. Just seeing the child happy is usually enough.

But as the children grow older, the loving parents begin to expect more from them; eventually, when we have given a lot, it is reasonable to expect something in return. When they don't get what they expect from the child, some couples begin to blame the other and, in doing so, reduce the amount of love they are willing to give each other, and the marriage is harmed. For this problem, and many other problems too numerous to cite here, the choice theory that we will begin to explain shortly can be very helpful.

Power: The Mystery of Marriage Is in Our Genes

As explained in Chapter 3, marriage is unique to human beings. And unlike survival, love and belonging, freedom, and even fun, all of which can be seen in lower animals, the need for power is unique to human beings. Animals may fight for a territory, to protect their young, or for a mate to pass on their genes, but they do not fight, as we do, just for the sake of power. And for having our way, or punishing another for disagreeing with us, there is no human relationship more contentious than marriage. Why this is so and how it can be avoided is the key to solving the mystery of marriage.

Driven by the need for power, human beings have been harming and killing other people who have not harmed them since Cain killed Abel. Most of us, however, are not concerned with the extremes of power that make the front page. Even though we would like to have more money or prestige, our power need generally is satisfied if we are respected.

To gain respect, the minimum needed is that someone we care about, ideally, our partner, listens to us. If we don't have that, at first we struggle to get it, but after a while most of us give up and don't even try to communicate seriously anymore, and the relationship is badly harmed. What we may do for power, if we decide to stay married, is to get most of our satisfaction from actively or passively struggling with our mate.

Our need for power makes it hard for us to accept a low-power position in any relationship, particularly a marriage. I believe that a huge obstacle to a happy marriage is the inability of one or both partners to satisfy their need for power in the partnership. It is rarely the lack of love that destroys relationships; it is more that long-term love cannot take root in a relationship in which one or both of the partners believe they have less power than they believe they need or want.

For any partnership to succeed, and marriage is no exception, the partners need to be friends, to be able to enjoy each other's company. Much more than sex and love, friendship is based on equal power or no power, and equal power is based on listening to each other, really paying attention. There is no other way. I see this need for power every day in my practice. Virtually every therapy client says over and over how empowering it is to talk to someone who actually listens and takes them seriously.

Power May Be the Genetic Origin of External Control Psychology

We believe that our need for power is the source of our universal practice of external control psychology. And as long as we use external control, we will kill enough marital happiness so that a long, happy marriage will continue to be the least attainable of all our long-term relationships. Since power is built into our genes, we have no chance of getting rid of it. But external control psychology is not built into our genes; like all else we do, it is chosen. This means that any couple who is willing to replace it in their marriage with choice theory has an excellent chance for a happy marriage. Carleen and I and many other couples we know have done this, so we know it can be done. Once a couple understands choice theory, most of the mysteries of marriage disappear.

In practice, choice theory teaches that you can control only your own behavior. No one can control you, and you can't control anyone else. But, you point out, some people—for example, the man you work for—can make you do a lot of things you don't want to do. My answer is that if you are willing to suffer the consequences, up to and including losing your life, no one can make you do anything you don't want to do. And even if you accept the control of others such as your boss, they can't control what you are thinking while you are doing it. Many a woman submits to her husband's sexual advances, but no woman can be forced to love her husband while she does it.

From Cheryl's letter and my meeting with Larry, I knew that their failing marriage was the embodiment of what happens when two external control people marry and stay together for twenty years. Because they practice external control, I also know that what they are asking us is to tell them how each can make the other change. We don't know exactly what Cheryl wants from Larry, but we do know that Larry wants Cheryl to stop her endless complaining. They both may have a vague idea that they can control only themselves, but in practice they really believe they can control the other—even though for twenty years they have not succeeded in doing so. And they are polished professionals in employing the seven deadly habits in their marriage.

Although the habits are all destructive, the first, criticizing, is the most destructive. That behavior alone wrecks a marriage, and it is the one most to be avoided if we are to have any chance for a happy marriage. If there is any love left in a marriage, stopping the destructive habits goes a long way toward reviving what seems to be close to dead. We are curious to see if Cheryl and Larry will give this a try. The key, however, is not only to stop using the habits but also to replace them with choice theory.

Freedom: The Need That Challenges Marriage

Freedom is ordinarily the desire to do what we want to do. In marriage, this means to get out from under the control of one's mate. In contrast to power, where we try to control others, here the difficult task is to give up something your genes strongly ask you not to give up. The very nature of marriage is loss of personal freedom. As a rule, people who have a low need for freedom are much happier in marriage than those with a higher need to be left alone. Much of the rage that erupts in marriage is caused by one partner, often the man, feeling too restricted.

When there is a problem with freedom, the only avenue that has a chance to work is negotiation. If some amount of freedom agreeable to both can't be negotiated, there can be no happiness in that marriage. It is not uncommon for couples who divorce to find short periods of happiness with each other now that they are no longer restricted by their marriage. Sometimes these couples are fooled by how well they get along in these brief get-togethers and make the mistake of remarrying, only to go through the same process again.

Negotiating freedom is perhaps the most difficult of all marital negotiations, and knowing how strong each partner's freedom need is before marriage should be taken into account. It may be possible for a woman to teach a man to be more loving, because the man feels better when he learns to do this. But to persuade a man that he will feel better when he gives up freedom is much more difficult. To ask people to give up more freedom than they are capable of giving is to ask them to suffer more pain than the marriage may be worth to them.

The only hope in this scenario is if the need for love and belonging overrides the need for freedom. People who are deeply in love gladly give each other freedom and feel secure enough in their love and within themselves to not resent giving each other the space they need. Emotional dependence is an external control behavior. Learning choice theory helps one understand how to fill one's own space when the other is not there.

Fun: The Need That Is Most Easily Satisfied in Marriage

Fun is a need that we can satisfy by ourselves or with others. It can be satisfied in so many ways, at so many places, and at almost any time of the day or night. Babies as young as six months can begin to have fun. The game of peekaboo is enjoyed by almost everyone who has a little baby, and the baby enjoys it as much as or more than the adult.

Unlike power but very much like survival, love, and freedom, fun is built into the genes of almost all animals. Young mammals such as dogs and cats seem to expend a lot of energy playing and appear to be trying to have fun. But as they mature, they revert mostly to the survival activities of eating, sleeping, and sex when in season. Animals in the wild also play when young, but when they mature, they stick pretty much to the business of survival, including sex. Their play seems to be a way they learn, and once they are mature they stop playing because they have learned all they need to know.

What I have concluded is that for mammals and maybe birds, fun is the genetic reward for the kind of play in which they have a chance to learn new ways to behave that they can use all their lives. The more evolved the animal, the longer it plays and the longer it learns. We humans learn all of our lives, so we play all of our lives. Driven by the need for fun, we carry play to an extreme far beyond that of any lower creature. For example, we engage in a lot of social play and even enjoy watching others play, as when we watch sports. Many who play devote a large amount of energy to trying to win.

But we strive for fun in many ways that have nothing to

do with playing or winning. Reading, listening to music, traveling, and engaging in hobbies all are fun activities. In fact, driven by our need for fun there is hardly a human activity that is not pursued for fun by those who want to do it better. Every one of these activities is also pursued for excellence as we try to improve by learning more. The whole process—improving, learning, and laughing—goes on and on.

It is obvious that people who can learn have a survival advantage over people who cannot learn or over people who can't learn as fast or as well. It is from this advantage that the need for fun became built into our genes. Just as we are the descendants of high-survival people who took loving care of their young, competed to pass along their genes, or struggled to be free of others who tried to dominate them, we are also descended from people who learned better than their neighbors.

It is also obvious from all the marital unhappiness that marriage, universal as it is, is not built into our genes. In our opinion, it is a practice in desperate need of improvement. So with all the reasons there are to try to improve it, another mystery of marriage is, *Why do so many people who enjoy fun in many other areas find so little fun in marriage?*

It strikes both Carleen and me that our marriage is filled with fun. Just for fun, we do many things together that we enjoy. It seems to us that to help their marriage, the one thing Cheryl and Larry could do that is easy and available in so many ways is to try to have more fun together. Fun doesn't require sex, money, great effort, or good health; all it requires is that they start doing again what they did so much of together, whatever it was, before they were married and early in their marriage. And to look into new activities that could still be a lot of fun. All that is stopping them is the external control psychology they have been practicing for years.

There is no greater obstacle to fun than criticizing, blaming, complaining, and nagging. We guess that at this stage of their marriage, the idea of having fun together doesn't even cross their minds. Here we have a genetic drive that is easy and enjoyable to satisfy, but almost all unhappy married couples ignore what could easily help them more than anything else.

Fun has great staying power. Sex and even love may wane over a long marriage, but fun remains fresh because, unlike sex, it can always go off in a new direction, and there are almost no restrictions on having fun. We all know people who have found an interest later in life that has transformed them. And many of these interests could be shared, at least to some extent, with a partner. Even if the partner does nothing more than show interest in what they are doing, they will have discovered one of the vital secrets of a long and happy marriage.

We have no intention of going through a list or a set of directions on how to have fun. If a couple like Cheryl and Larry are not able to get involved with what we suggest here and have some fun together, there is little we can offer that will help their relationship. It is also important that they not get involved in trying to figure out if they need to get rid of external control to have fun. They don't have to do anything but try to have some fun together. As soon as they start, they immediately reduce their use of external control. And the more they reduce it, the more fun is possible. Fun is the most certain win-win activity of marriage. We hope they will take advantage of it.

Choice Theory

Basically, choice theory explains that the only person we can control is ourselves. If we are dissatisfied in a relationship, we should focus on what we can do to improve the relationship and not attempt to change the other. The partner almost always changes as we rid ourselves of external control. But choice theory goes beyond ridding ourselves of external control. It says we should do all we can to make it as easy as possible for our partner to satisfy his or her needs. To do this we should start substituting what I call the seven caring habits of choice theory: (1) *listening*, (2) *supporting*, (3) *encouraging*, (4) *respecting*, (5) *trusting*, (6) *accepting*, and (7) *always negotiating disagreements*.

The power of choice theory is that it helps us to get along with other people, especially with the people close to us. In our experience, it is the only way to maintain a long-term, happy marriage. What we do when we practice choice theory when we have even an inkling of a problem is to think before we deal with each other. The first thing we think about is avoiding using the seven deadly habits, because we know they will separate us further and increase the problem.

Next we make sure that we use one or more of the seven caring habits as we attempt to deal with our differences. As simple as this seems, it is almost impossible to do unless you recognize how much harm you are doing to your marriage with the deadly habits. Once a word comes out of your mouth or an expression crosses your face, you can't retract it. And while the habits don't actually drive your partner away, it is almost totally predictable that he or she will choose to withdraw further from you than he or she is now.

The only way to deal with any marital conflict is to negotiate using caring language or the language of choice theory. The success of marriage is directly proportional to how well the couple learns to negotiate. And the success of a marital negotiation depends on how well both parties in the negotiation understand the most basic of all the choice-theory concepts: *We can control only our own behavior.* Most of what is called negotiation in the real world is firmly rooted in external control. For example, I would try to convince you how much less you would suffer if you accepted my offer. And you would try to do the same to me. Please note: I wrote *to* me, not *for* me.

A choice-theory negotiation, on the other hand, is based on what each party can offer that he or she believes would help solve the problem. It is what is commonly called a win-win negotiation. In real estate, a simple win-win negotiation is I want $100,000 for my house, you offer $80,000, and we agree that $90,000 is fair to both of us. Neither of us got all we wanted, but we got an amount we thought was fair and settled. Unlike most real-world negotiations, neither of us tried to pressure the other to give us more than our fair share.

In marriage, a choice-theory negotiation might be that the wife wants her husband to come home every night for dinner. He says he can't come home every night or he'll lose his job. Using external control, she keeps nagging, and he works even later both to spite her and to avoid her nagging. They then learn choice theory, and he offers to come home two nights one week and three nights the next at a minimum. She accepts his offer as fair and agrees to stop nagging. He enjoys getting rid of the nagging so much that he begins to show up more often in the week.

This may sound simple, but it is exactly what works to help the marriage.

Committed naggers might insist that if she didn't nag, he would never come home. She had to nag to get what she wanted. But that argument is from the standpoint of external control. Once they use choice theory, that doesn't happen. She gets some, but not all she wants, but they both get a lot more love and joy, which more than makes up for his having to work some nights. As stated earlier, communication is vital, but as soon as it gets difficult, the best thing to replace it with is negotiation.

6

Sex After Marriage

In the movie *Sleeper,* Woody Allen plays a man who wakes up after being asleep for two hundred years. Someone asks him when he last had sex. He thinks awhile and replies, "Two hundred years ago." Then he pauses, thinks some more, and says, "Two hundred and six if you include my marriage." This humor typifies the general attitude about sex after marriage: less often and less exciting.

Sex and desire after marriage are, essentially, absent from movies, books, plays, and operas. And from the standpoint of audience interest, adulterous sex is by far the most popular. In Cheryl and Larry's marriage, this theme is confirmed. Sex with each other is minimal. What Cheryl does out of marriage is not known, but adultery with married women has been Larry's major sexual activity for years.

There is a whole host of research that attempts to document the general decline of sexual activity after ten years of marriage. The basic conclusions are that sex continues but at a much lower rate, once or twice a week. But the research does not show how satisfying the sex is or whether it ever approaches the urgent, desirable sex that begins most marriages. We believe that this drop-off in postmarital sexual desire is closely linked to the use of external control psychology by one or both partners on the other. Nothing kills sex faster and more completely than the seven deadly habits.

For sex to work, the male has to be able to perform. Unlike women, men can't fake it. Perhaps the most distressing part of being a husband who wants to continue good sex after marriage is concern about his performance. Not each time, but still often enough to be distressing, the thought *Will I be able to perform this time well enough to satisfy both of us?* runs through the husband's mind. Once this thought gains entry, it is almost impossible to dispel it.

Many married men deal with that concern by refraining from sex, kind of *nothing ventured, nothing lost*. His wife may sense his distress, but she usually doesn't know how to cope with it, and neither of them wants to talk about it. From her standpoint, the best option may be to become passive and accepting, because becoming demanding will increase his performance concern. Many men wait until their prostates are so packed with seminal fluid that their ability to perform is physically enhanced, a wait that adds to the decline in frequency. However, the problem with waiting too long is premature ejaculation, which is distressing to the man and frustrating to the woman. From the woman's standpoint, waiting often is not a problem, but when he finally does it she wants it done well.

If a husband is to have the confidence that he can perform successfully with the same partner year after year, he needs to give his wife loving support and encouragement. If her life is hectic, she needs patient and loving foreplay to let her know he cares. What he needs from her if he is to gain the confidence that he can succeed are a lot of compliments on his performance during and after the act. And if he occasionally fails, a large amount of love, support, and encouragement all aimed at telling him he's okay, no one's perfect at everything. But especially, no criticism. If she criticizes, he may become impotent, which, in a hostile marriage filled with external control, may be exactly what she wants. If they can't do what is suggested here and a lot more that they can figure out on their own, they can forget about satisfying sex. Sex after marriage is complicated; if it is to succeed, it needs a lot of love both in and out of bed.

To maintain the confidence a man needs to perform well year after year, it is important that his wife be willing to tell him what she wants. This is not only good for her, it is especially good for him. It gives him something he can succeed in doing that has no chance of failure. And as he satisfies her, his confidence increases and he gets sex more and more on his mind. If she won't tell him what she wants, he should make the effort to figure it out, or figure out a way he can ask her if she isn't the kind to come out and tell him what she wants. But if he does what she wants in a very loving, patient way, he has a right to expect that, within reason, she will do the same for him.

The main impetus by far for both married men and women who engage in long-term affairs is the attempt to recapture the intimacy, sexual and personal, that they no longer find in their marriage. This was clear in Larry's description of how he conducts these activities. Therefore, in affairs that work—and all affairs work for a while or they wouldn't begin in the first place—it is because neither partner *criticizes, blames, complains, or nags*. Because they have to be with each other for only short periods of time, they accept the other for who he or she is and don't ask for more. The affair ends as soon as any of the deadly habits surface, which they often do. That doesn't mean affairs don't end for other reasons, but if the habits show up, they kill the intimacy and the affair is over.

Unfortunately, as long as we have external control psychology, affairs will have a sexual advantage over marriage that is hard for marriage to compete with. For sex to be both desirable and successful, in or out of marriage, making love, *not defending and attacking each other*, has to be very much on the minds of both partners, at least for a while before they go to bed and exclusively as they begin to make love.

Wives and husbands tend to use what they know, the deadly habits. But besides the habits, they also have a myriad of things on their minds besides sex. For example, things you would never say to your illicit partner you may say to your spouse, even in the bedroom, such as: *Please take a look at the toilet, I think it's running*, or any other of a dozen concerns such as money, children, school, parents, or bosses that may be on the minds of couples. These concerns are very hard to suspend before and even during sex.

In fact, one of the great mysteries of marriage is this sexual decline. Is it because sex no longer feels good? I doubt that. A major concern of many married couples who are getting along well is that sex doesn't seem as important as it used to be. Sometimes they think it may be something physical, but it rarely is. What is usually wrong is nothing more than the fact that sex is just not on their minds as much as it used to be and as much as it needs to be for it to be successful. Married couples have told me that when they get around to doing it, it's still good, but they just don't seem to get around to doing it often enough to keep it on their minds.

To this end, I'd like to relate what was told to me by a woman who came to see me because of problems with her aging mother. She wanted some advice on how to move her once independent mother into assisted living.

She was an attractive woman who by her demeanor seemed very aware of her appearance. She told me her mother was now eighty-six, so I judged her to be in her mid-fifties, but she looked no more than forty-five. These days it's difficult to tell a woman's age. After we discussed how to deal with her mother, we still had half an hour left and, as I usually do with clients, I asked her about the relationships in her own life.

I asked her because, in my experience, many people who come for help begin by presenting a problem about someone else, as she did with her mother, to kind of check me out. But what they really want to talk about is a current relationship problem, usually their marriage. It turned out she didn't have another problem. She actually had a success story she wanted to tell. She had solved the problem I've been discussing in this chapter: how to enjoy frequent and satisfying marital sex.

She told me, "I've been married for thirty-five years to a good man. When we got married we were very much in love and really hot for each other all the time. But then we had children, busy careers, he was immersed in starting what is now a successful printing business, and until recently I worked right alongside him. Then one day about five years ago I took stock of myself. I said to myself, '*Martha, what do you really want right now?*'"

"That's interesting. I don't think you know much about me"—she shook her head to say she didn't—"but that's the question I often ask the people who come to see me. I think it's a very good question. I ask it of myself once in a while."

I just looked at her to see what her answer would be.

"I don't know if anyone has ever told you this, but what I wanted was simple. I wanted more sex. It had all but disappeared in our marriage, to the point where neither of us seemed to be willing to do anything about it. It was like riding our bikes. For years we rode together, but then we stopped and our bikes have just hung there in the garage gathering dust. It's as if what was once an important part of our life had been suspended, kind of put on hold, and neither of us had any idea how to get it going again."

I looked at her and she continued. "I read the advice columns, and they talk about sex therapy. I read catalogs, and they talk about mechanical aids like vibrators. And now all the hullabaloo about Viagra. None of that stuff made much sense to me. There was nothing wrong with us physically, we'd done it many times, and I didn't see any need for sex therapy. I didn't want to talk about sex. I wanted to *do* it and not just once. I can still get him to do it once in a while, but I wanted it more than that. I wanted him to be hot for me. And I hated to nag him about it. I even thought about having an affair, but no one in our circle looked any better to me than he did. I wanted him to want me and to be interested in doing it. To act like a young man because, Doctor, what I wanted was a young man. I still feel every inch a young woman."

"You must have succeeded or you wouldn't have brought it up."

"Succeeded is putting it mildly. That man is as horny as a goat, and I love it. But what I'm proud of is I figured out it was my problem. If I wanted him to act like a young man, I had to begin acting like a young woman."

"Okay, please tell me what you did. It's not often I get someone in here with a success story. All I hear is people complaining about their lives."

"The first thing I thought of was to do some research, so I sent away for videotapes. Not the clinical ones they advertise in health magazines. The kind they advertise in *Penthouse* and magazines like that. I'd heard about them, but I'd never seen one. Sure enough, just as they said in the ads, a plain brown paper package came to the house. I'm home now all the time. He goes to our business every day, so he didn't see what came in the package. There was a reduced price if you bought a dozen, so that's what I did. Then I started to watch them, and I'll tell you, those tapes got me excited. I hadn't had those feelings for a very long time."

She paused a moment to kind of ponder what she was saying. Then with a tiny smile on her face, she went on.

"I waited until Sunday morning. He plays golf every Sunday, ten-thirty tee time, and he always wakes up in a good mood. Around eight, I got up to go to the john. Then before I got back into bed I took off my nightgown, and when I got under the covers I snuggled up to him. He could feel I was naked, but he had his mind on golf and didn't say anything. I said to him, 'You know what? I feel like watching television, would you like to watch with me?' Well, we never watch television in the morning, and we've had a set and a VCR in our bedroom for twenty years. So he said, 'What's gotten into you? You hardly ever look at TV. I don't think you've ever watched it before breakfast. What's going on?' I said, 'It's not television, it's a videotape. I bought a few and I'd like to show you one. I've watched it alone, but I said to myself, that's no fun, I bet Paul would like to watch this one with me. You see, it's about this guy going to play golf.' He perked up.

"I got up and slowly went to the VCR and put in a tape. He's seen me naked before, but I don't think he's ever seen me put in a videotape quite the way I did without my clothes on—or for that matter with them on. He always works the machine, records football games and all that stuff on ESPN. I took a long time putting the tape in the VCR so he could see me like that awhile, and then, after it was all set and rolling, I turned around slowly with my hands on my hips and a smile on my face. Then, like a naughty little kitten, I crawled back under the covers beside him. The tape came on. But first we had to sit through all that free speech stuff with the flag flying and the national anthem playing. I just waited and watched the funny look he had on his face. I could sense he was getting aroused. Then the show began. I just snuggled up and watched with him. I think he's seen those tapes before. He goes to men's functions for business, but he's never seen them with me, and it was obvious he was getting very interested in what was going on. Sure enough, there was a guy in his bedroom all decked out for golf in knickers with his clubs in a golf bag, the whole nine yards. And there was this woman, I guess it was his wife, in bed. Her shtick was to try to get him to stay home with her. She goes through her whole act, he stays home and they play. I just stayed there beside Paul, and we watched until they finished. Then I reached down to make sure he was interested, and he certainly was. So I turned off the VCR with the remote, tore the covers off the bed, and said, 'Paul, honey, I want to do to you right now everything that woman did to the man on the tape. You don't have to do anything at all, just lie on your back and relax.' And I did. But he didn't relax. I was afraid he couldn't last and I wanted him to so I had to stop and start a couple of times. It was driving him crazy. Every time he made a move for me, I slapped his hand and said, 'No, not yet.' Then when I was sure he was really interested, I said, 'Now, I'd like you to do to me just what that guy did to her. But only if you want to. If you don't or this bothers you, just tell me.'

"Well, that's the story. I don't have to tell you what happened—plenty did. The old man actually did it twice. He hadn't done that since our honeymoon. He was just as surprised as I was, and I had to push him out of bed to go play golf. At breakfast I told him if it was okay with him we could do that whenever we felt like it from now on. I had a dozen tapes and at a half hour at a time, they'd last for months. Actually, the way he's been they'll last forever. All they did was get him started, sort of prime the pump, so to speak. He's been going strong on his own now for over five years. Doctor, this may be the best sex of our marriage. When he got home from golf, I asked him if he'd told his buddies about what'd happened. He looked at me as if I was crazy. He asked me if I was going to tell anyone. Teasing, I said, 'Just your mother. Can't I tell her the boy she raised is quite a man?'"

I saw Martha a few more times about her mother, and she never mentioned sex again. But I kept thinking that she did something creative, something that anyone with a stale marriage could do. And when we decided to write this book, I thought that incident fit here perfectly. Obviously his real name's not Paul and hers is not Martha, and she came to see me for a reason other than her mother.

By telling you about Martha and Paul, I'm not in any way suggesting that all a couple needs to do is watch some porno flicks and that will save their crumbling marriage. I am merely pointing out that as an alternative to a stale and sexless existence, couples can be creative. In this case, Martha was the creative one, but it could very well have been her husband doing something to spark the marriage. The way we look at it, all we have going for us as men and women, in it for the duration, is our cleverness and our willingness to try something else when what we're doing isn't working. But no amount of creativity will help a sagging sex life if you refuse to give up using external control on each other.

Finally, I think that combining all the marital sex inhibitors explained in this chapter with our general distrust of sex, which is a part of our puritan heritage, people enter marriage with what we call lowered sexual priorities. By that I mean that as the marriage continues, a whole host of marital concerns take precedence over sex. It's as if we can always have sex, so it can wait; there are so many other things we have to do first. But like everything else we do, this lowered priority is a choice.

Couples don't have to lower their sex priorities. In fact, we strongly believe that couples should make every effort to raise their expectations of sex after marriage. This is the time to get creative and try to figure out a way to have sex as often as possible for as long as the couple is married.

Sexual pleasure is one of nature's great offerings. To throw it away as so many couples do is to refuse to accept one of the greatest gifts our genes have bestowed upon us.

At this point we are ready to send the first six chapters of this book to Cheryl and Larry. Both Carleen and I are very interested in what they will do with this information.

7

Feedback

About a month went by before we got a reply, first from Larry and then from both of them, to the first six chapters we sent. The following is Larry's e-mail.

> Thank you very much for the chapters. We both read them very carefully, and Cheryl will be sending you our first feedback in a few weeks. To say that we saw our whole marriage unfold in these chapters is to understate the impact they had on us. So much on me, that I want to ask another favor of you, and I'm counting on you to keep this e-mail confidential and not refer to it if you write to Cheryl.
>
> The woman I am presently having an affair with is named Ellen, and we share our lives with each other. I don't mean that we talk in detail about our marriages, but we are both interested in doing as much for each

other as we can. I talked to Ellen about what you sent us, and she is also interested in reading it to see if it applies to her marriage. I know you gave us permission to share it, but I still wanted to check with you because what she wants to do is different from us. She promises to keep it confidential, and I believe she can be trusted.

Here is what she proposes to do. In our case, Cheryl and I are working together on these ideas. Ellen can't do that. She has no idea how to tell her husband where she got the information, and she has no assurance he'd be interested in doing with her what Cheryl and I are trying to do with each other. What she wants to do is use the ideas in her marriage but not tell him what she's doing, and then share what happened with you. I can see no reason for her not to, but unless you give me permission, I won't do it.

I would think that for you the advantage of her doing this is obvious. If the book is to succeed, it should be able to be used by one partner effectively even if the other partner is not aware of what he or she is doing—or not immediately aware of it. I've thought a lot about the material, and I see no reason why this wouldn't be possible. In fact, I am already trying to ratchet up the fun in our marriage based on your explanation of that basic need without telling Cheryl, and it seems to be working. Martha, the videotape lady, did what she did without consulting her husband, and it seemed to work.

Since you are disguising all the characters, Ellen said it would be fine with her to use in your book anything she does that helped her marriage. To give me the go-ahead on this request, just leave a message on my answering machine at the office and say you accept my proposal for Ellen. You don't have to leave your name.

Thanks,
Larry

Carleen and I agreed that there was no reason to turn down Larry's request. So now we are looking forward to getting feedback from Ellen as well, and as Larry said, it could be valuable. We have been teaching choice theory long enough to know that it can be effective for a while if only one person in a relationship begins to use it.

About three and a half weeks after Larry sent the e-mail about Ellen, we got our first communication from Larry and Cheryl.

Dear Bill and Carleen,

We hope you excuse our use of your first names, but it seems right to us that we should all be on a first-name basis. Bill, as you do in your book, I will be the primary writer so the pronoun "I" refers to me, Cheryl. But Larry will read and approve of what I write, and when he has something he especially wants to say, he'll use his name.

Needless to say, those chapters have been a revelation, and we have been talking every day about how we should use that information. As you may suspect, our marriage is already better, because where we had little or no real communication for years, now we are talking all the time. We have agreed that while everything you explain is useful, there are three things in particular that we are trying to do right now: get rid of the seven deadly habits, implement the need for fun, and try to get more love and sex back into our relationship. Let's start with the habits.

First of all, I have always been aware that I'm a world-class complainer, and that Larry has to listen to it endlessly every day. I really wonder why he came home at all some days knowing he had to face my barrage of what's wrong with the world. Why I do this or when it started is immaterial. Neither of us is into pop psychology with all its explanations aimed at blaming others for the way we choose to screw up our lives. Notice, I'm using the word *choose*. We are both starting to use that word. It really clears up what's been a flood of muddy water.

After learning about the habits, Larry admits to being a know-it-all and a criticizer. He gets a big kick out of putting his students down with his "superior" knowledge, and he's trying to stop it. While he doesn't criticize me as openly as he does everything and everybody else, nonetheless I hear a lot of criticism of me in his put-downs of others just as he hears a lot of "it's his fault" in so many of my complaints. While we were both mildly aware of what we were doing, it wasn't until we saw it in black and white in your chapters that we were both willing to admit that what we'd been doing for years was killing our marriage.

But it's one thing to recognize it and another to get rid of it. Lifelong habits don't just melt away. But now when it happens, instead of getting all bent out of shape, we admit it and talk about it. And best of all, we laugh about it. I stop myself in mid sentence and say, "I've got to say this. I just have to, so I will." But then I say, "At least I recognize what I'm doing and I'm trying to stop." Larry says we're like alcoholics with AA. We're recovering external control freaks. But we've got a way to go and don't expect miracles. But the good thing is, all the malice and anger are gone from what we say. We just laugh and try to stop.

What I do instead of complaining is try to do something about it. But usually I can't do anything to remedy the situation, so now, following choice theory, I accept that the only person's behavior I can control is my own. For example, I used to go on for hours and hours about the parents of the kids in my nursery school, but now I say to myself, "They're not perfect, and it's their problem, not mine." As soon as he got home, Larry'd rush to turn on the television to drown me out. I'm slowly beginning to accept that all I can do is take good care of their kids, meet with parents when they want to meet with me, but stop trying to control what they do with their kids like I used to.

Larry says we definitely have the habits on the run. What amazes me is that it's so simple. What we do now when we have a problem is take your advice and negotiate. We're finding that if we say only what each one of us can do to help and leave the other to say the same, almost everything gets worked out. Getting rid of the habits and negotiating the differences between us is a real confirmation of what you and Carleen are trying to teach.

As we got rid of the habits, we slowly began to accept that we're in this marriage for the duration. And if we're locked together, what sense does it make to do things that harm each other? You can't possibly harm the other without harming yourself, can you? We keep thinking of the fable about the scorpion and the turtle. Remember, the scorpion wants to cross the river and asks the turtle to ferry him across. The turtle says he's frightened that the scorpion will sting him on the way over and kill him. But the scorpion says, "Why would I do that? If I sting you and kill you, I'll drown, too. There's nothing for you to fear." It made sense to the turtle, so he agreed to take him. But halfway across, the scorpion stings the turtle and wounds him critically. As he begins to sink, the turtle asks the scorpion why he did it. "Now you're going to drown, too." He says, "I couldn't help it, it's my nature." Well, external control was our nature, but finally, after all these years, we have a little more sense than the scorpion.

Okay, so far we're getting the habits under control. But we know this may just be a honeymoon period; it may fade away and we may go back to being scorpions. Larry says we have to watch everything we do and say for a long time, and I agree. You can't believe how easily a complaint slips out of my mouth. But, as I said, at least I recognize it when I hear it. It's not difficult if we make a joke about it. Humor detoxifies external control. Larry had a great sense of humor when we got married, but he stopped using it around me. Now I'm encouraging him to use it again. I even encourage him to make fun of me when I slip back into complaining. He's figured out some funny ways to deal with me when I slip. He compliments me for trying and tells me he appreciates what we're both trying to do.

Okay, now I guess it's time to talk to you about sex. You were right when you said that men worry about failure, and quite a while ago Larry began to fail with me. Not every time, but it didn't take more than a few times to get him discouraged. And as soon as he got worried about whether he would be able to finish what he started, he couldn't even get started. And when he did succeed, he suffered from premature ejaculation, which I guess is just another form of failure. I didn't put him down or act dissatisfied, but it didn't seem to help. We never talked about it, and our sex life almost disappeared. But when we read the chapter on sex in the book, I learned a lot, and so did he. And best of all, we talked about it, and that was the first time since we've known each other that he's been able to talk to me about sex. Keep in mind that Larry's aware of and approves of what I'm writing here.

Now here's the point. You talked extensively about the difference between sex in marriage and sex in affairs. You explained that many men and women are able to have better sex in affairs because of a variety of reasons such as no external control in an affair, and, in an affair, sex is front and center on both partners' minds. After I read that chapter, I began to think that maybe he'd lost interest in me after a few failures because he was having an affair. Or he began to have an affair and then didn't even want to make it work with me.

But more and more that chapter made it hard for me to believe that a man as young as Larry—he's only forty-six and I'm forty-two—who had been as sexual as he was in the beginning, would give up on sex as easily as he had with me. I mean, if we did it once a month it was a big deal for him. But then I asked myself, "If he's been having an affair or a series of affairs, and I'm well aware of the fact that college professors are notoriously promiscuous, do I really want to know?" And then the thought occurred to me that if I'd been having an affair, would he really want to know? So about a week ago, I brought this subject up.

I said, "In Chapter Six, they suggest that sex drops off after marriage, and ours certainly has. I also read about affairs in that chapter, and if you've been having an affair or affairs, I can see why you've been doing it. That doesn't make it right or excuse it, but I'm perfectly willing to accept that this may be what's been going on even though I don't like it. It would certainly explain why we have had so little sex for so many years. Without you admitting anything, because either way I don't want to know, will you agree with me that what Dr. Glasser wrote in that chapter is reasonable?"

Larry thought for a moment and said, "It's very reasonable, all of it. Affairs have been a part of academia since the beginning of time. They go on between staff and staff and between staff and students and, today, very few students are sexually inactive if they have any chance to be otherwise."

I said to Larry, "Otherwise is such a pretentious word, and this is such a heavy subject. Do you mind if I lighten it up a little?"

He said, "Be my guest."

So I said, "I think it's only fair for me to answer the same question I asked you about that chapter on affairs. Would that be okay with you if I did?" He said that yes it would. "Larry, has it ever crossed your mind that a good-looking, forty-two-year-old woman like me, who used to like sex and who isn't getting any at home, might have been having an affair or two herself over the past ten years?"

Very quickly, without any hesitation he said, "Truthfully, that possibility's never crossed my mind."

"So, if I have or you have or we both have or are still having affairs, would it be okay if we never get into that area in our discussions about our marriage?"

Then before he realized what he was saying, he said, "Cheryl, are you intimating that you could have been having affairs all these years?"

Then I said, and I could see the surprise on his face, "I certainly could be. But I'm also asking if it's all right with you if I don't confess. Because I have no intention of confessing about anything in my whole life prior to today. And I have no interest in hearing a confession from you about anything that happened before today in your life. Can you live with this? Because if you can't, I think we're going to have trouble getting our marriage going again. And I want nothing more than to try to get it going. I want to start over, with a clean slate. If I've been having affairs or you've been having affairs, I'd like both of us to use what we've learned to treat each other better than before. Why squander our riches elsewhere? For my part, I'd like to go sexy Martha from Chapter Six one better. I'd like to pretend we're making our own videotapes, if that's okay with you?"

So that's what we're doing. Do you think we're catching on, or are we misreading what you wrote? Don't bother to write if you think we're on the right track.

Love,
Larry and Cheryl

Carleen and I talked about that e-mail for a long time. First of all we decided that they were definitely on the right track. We also talked about the fact that we knew what Larry was doing and we wondered from what Cheryl said if she knew. And we also wondered if she had been having affairs. There was certainly a little male chauvinism in Larry's concern about Cheryl's potential for extramarital activities. Carleen said she thought that Cheryl was doing the only thing that had a chance of working in that tenuous situation: trying to make a fresh start. You can't undo the past no matter what happened or how hard you try.

I said that I appreciated what Cheryl did. I was wondering how we were going to write an honest book knowing what we knew about Larry. And yet, we had no right to betray his disclosure. But Carleen said he'd done a pretty good job of betraying it himself with that sudden concern about what she might have been doing. I guess the gander takes a chance when he begins to see what's good for the goose.

Still, we both wondered how readers of the book would deal with what she did. I think many of them will think she was too forgiving. If she had any real suspicions, she should have had it out with him. But then we thought, if she had, she might have won the battle but she would have lost the war. There'd be no chance they could breathe life back into their marriage after that kind of a blowup. What she did, we agreed, was liberating. She freed herself from the burden of trying to monitor his behavior and chose to control the only person she can control, herself.

We also got into a discussion about whether he was worth taking back. But Cheryl is the only one who can make that decision, so our discussion was purely academic. It's her life. If she wants to take a chance on him, it's no one's business but her own. When we start making moral decisions for other people, when no one can get hurt except the people involved, we're about as deep into external control as you can get.

The final question we asked ourselves is, Will this improvement last, or will it just be temporary? That question cannot be answered. No one can predict human behavior. All we can say is that from where they were when Cheryl first e-mailed me to where they seem to be now, their marriage is already a lot better. We are also heartened by the fact that they not only understood what we were saying but also were able to put it to work in their lives.

We still have a way to go. We have some more to say in this book, and we expect to hear from Cheryl and Larry again. We also hope to hear from Ellen. It will be interesting to see if Larry stops seeing Ellen, or if she stops seeing him. Will they talk it over and decide to stop seeing each other and try to make a go of their own marriages?

8

Our Quality World Confirms Our Love

Choice theory teaches that we all have what we call a quality world: a detailed, precise simulation of a special world we would like to live in if we could. While it occupies only a tiny portion of our memory, we believe it's the core of our life. Created, starting at birth, and continually re-created until we die, it contains pictures of our most pleasurable need-satisfying activities and is the source of all our specific motivation. The memory pictures we store in it feature people, including a constantly changing picture of ourselves, objects such as prized possessions, and systems of belief such as our deepest and most cherished religious tenets. It is called a world because it represents an ideal world, for each of us our personal Shangri-la.

As long as we live, the pictures in our quality world are the actual motivation for all our behavior. While the needs are the genetic source, it is these very specific pictures of the way we want to live our lives that cause us to do whatever we do from birth to death. For example, when Cheryl and Larry got married, Cheryl's quality world contained a picture of Larry happily married to her along with a picture of her happily married to him. The equivalent pictures of her and him were in his quality world.

In each of their minds, there was a strong hope that, as the marriage continued, they would find ways to treat each other that would continue to satisfy those initial pictures. But this is precisely what they—and many couples—had been unable to do. While our quality world contains pictures of what we want, it is our task to figure out how to behave to keep those pictures satisfied. If we are unable to figure out how to do this, the behaviors we choose to try to do it become more and more painful. Cheryl complains and Larry criticizes; neither behavior is even remotely satisfying to what they still picture in their quality worlds.

At this point they, and all other couples with failing marriages, have three choices. First, they can stay married and continue to keep those initial pictures in their quality world, all the while knowing that what they are doing has no chance of satisfying them. If they do this, their suffering will continue to be acute. Second, one or both of them can modify the picture of each other and of themselves to expect little more from each other than that they stay married. This reduces but does not eliminate the pain. (This is what Cheryl and Larry had chosen to do, but it didn't work well. It also prompted Cheryl's letter to us.) Third, one or both of them can take the other out of his or her quality world. For the one who takes the other's picture out, the pain is lessened. If they both take the other out, they both get relief from the pain. Whether they then divorce or not, the marriage is essentially over.

Few people realize the power their quality world has over their lives. As long as we keep a picture in it and fail to satisfy that picture, we suffer. There is no escape from that reality; it is the way our brain works. But the good part is that our quality world is sacrosanct to us in the sense that we have total control over what goes into it, what changes are made in it, and what is taken out of it. It has no morality, no sense of right or wrong as the real world sees right or wrong. And no matter what we say or protest, it is what we see in our quality world as right, or moral, that is the source of our actual morality. The rest is wishful thinking.

What I've just explained makes it sound easy to change: If what we want is hard to get, just stop wanting it. But of course this is almost never the case. We put it in our quality world because it was, or we believed it to be, a great source of pleasure. If we take it out, we are admitting that we have given up on regaining that pleasure. This is what Cheryl and Larry don't want to do. It is also what many couples, if not most couples, married or not, don't want to do. Even though they are not happy with their marriage or relationship, they don't want to give up on it because they can't envision their quality world without marriage in it.

Carleen and I are in each other's quality world as husband and wife. In my quality world, I picture myself doing things that please her and her doing things that please me. I do not picture myself using any of the seven deadly habits on her, and I hope she pictures herself never using the seven deadly habits on me.

But I have control over only what I picture. I have no control over what she pictures. Yet I know that the better I treat her, the better she treats me and the stronger we appear in each other's quality world. She in my quality world, and I in hers, confirm our love for each other. While we know only what is in our own quality world, one of the tests of our love is our willingness to share our quality worlds, she with me, I with her. The more completely each of us is willing to share this world, the more in love we become.

Sometime, usually early in our adolescence, driven strongly but not exclusively by the sex hormones generated by our need to survive, we begin to form an idea of who would make an ideal mate. From this early idea, a picture of this person begins to take shape in our quality world. For boys it may be a picture with some of the qualities of their mother; for girls, their father.

But driven by the popular media, we also begin to add to this ideal picture what we like about characters from movies, television, magazines, and books, as well as from relatives, neighbors, teachers, and friends. For almost all of us, this romanticizing continues most of our lives; it even wanders in and out of our minds when we are happily married. The less happy we are in our marriage, the more we fantasize about other people, and the more we get involved with other people, as Larry and Ellen became involved with each other.

Unfortunately, for many of us this picture is highly idealized or romanticized and bears little resemblance to who actually is available to marry. In marriage, "the honeymoon is over" is the pop phrase for the difference between the idealized person we hoped was our mate and the real person who, shortly after the marriage, we "discover" is our mate.

What we can learn from choice theory is that we alone

have control over the picture we put into our quality world, and that it makes sense to try to fall in love with someone who is realistic and available. Again, easy to say but hard to do. Still, if we don't understand the workings of our quality world, we may stray too far from who is real and, in doing so, deeper into misery.

Most of us are aware that the quality world picture of our mate when we marry is not realistic, and many of us are able to change that picture to adjust to the reality of who we married. But the more we have to do this, the more our marriage is challenged. Still, too many of us delude ourselves into believing that, *given our love,* our prospective partner can be changed into the idealized picture of him or her that we have placed in our quality world. More marital misery is caused by the shattering of this delusion than almost anything else we experience.

Although mates do change, in most instances they change in a direction a lot different from what we want. As we try to control our mates through the use of the seven habits so that they become closer to what we want, they resist, and if we persist, we will destroy our marriage. Here the choice-theory axiom, *We can change only ourselves,* applies strongly. Too many of us are blinded by what we want, and this blindness does not allow us to take into account what others want or are willing to do for us.

Therefore, although we can't control another person's quality world, we can continually try to find out what is in it and behave in a way that satisfies those pictures. The best guide to what our mate wants is the golden rule, "Do unto others as you would have others do unto you."

The most common way to try to control our mate that results from our use of the seven habits is to withdraw love and attention, as Cheryl and Larry did, from each other. As they did this, they grew farther apart. Cheryl and Larry are a good example of a couple whose marriage has stabilized some distance away from what either wants. In many instances, marriages don't stabilize, and the couple divorce. And once divorced, many men and women repeat the process, and a second or third marriage ends like the first.

But when a marriage becomes unhappy, if both the husband and the wife know about their quality worlds, they can use this knowledge to improve their marriage. For example, Cheryl and Larry can go beyond what they are now doing to help their marriage. First of all, they can admit to each other that they have changed their picture of each other to expect much less than they did when they got married. They should talk it over and admit that this is what has happened, and then tell each other that they would both like to improve the one picture they have in their quality world that they can change. *This is my picture of how I treat you. As much as I would like to, I can't change your picture of how you treat me.*

But they had also decided, when they contacted us, that they wanted to improve their marriage. This should mean that they can agree on a picture of marriage that is much better than the one they have now in their quality worlds. Then, if they can agree on what this better marriage looks like, they should each tell the other one specific thing each is willing to do all this coming week that he or she believes would improve their marriage.

For example, since they both work but both like to eat at home, and Larry isn't a cook—Cheryl loves to cook—Larry agrees to help with the food shopping and do the major cleanup after dinner. Cheryl offers to expand her menu to include more of Larry's favorites. They would share this offer with each other and, if the other agrees, they would each work hard to do it. But they would also agree that no matter what the other does, each will try to finish out the week doing what he or she promised to do. What each promised does not depend on the other doing his or her part; this is no quid pro quo. In choice-theory terms, they would not attempt to control the other.

This is because what they are doing is not for each other. It is for what they agreed would help their marriage. And if this suggestion works, it is because, in using it, they have agreed that their marriage takes precedence over what each wants for himself or herself. Anytime they help their marriage, they are helping themselves. For many couples this will be a first, but if they do it, they will raise their marriage to another level.

If Cheryl and Larry can keep doing this, by slowly adding to what they did the first week for several more weeks, they can help their marriage a great deal. But they must be tolerant. If one fails to do his or her share for a day or two, the other should keep going. And after a while they may suggest to the other what they need from each other, but only as a suggestion. No use of the deadly habits if the other doesn't do it. And no use of the habits if what the other tries in good faith doesn't work.

For years, Cheryl and Larry have had a picture of their marriage in their quality worlds that they weren't satisfying. The more they didn't get it, the more their marriage suffered. They may also have had many good ideas over the years of what each could do for the other, but when one tried, the other complained or criticized, so it didn't work and they gave up on it. But the flaw was that they were doing it for the other. What we are suggesting here is that they start doing it for their marriage, not for each other. This is different information, and we are anxious to see what they do with it after we send them the next set of chapters. Finally, when people are deeply in love, they trust each other enough to share almost their entire quality world, excluding what they are sure will hurt the other. A person would not share information about an affair, even after it ended. That is asking too much of another's love.

The more we are willing to share our quality worlds with each other, the more we love each other. But there is a risk in this sharing. Our quality world has our hopes, our wildest dreams, our most hidden aspirations, our most cherished beliefs deep inside it. If I open all this up to you, I become more vulnerable than ever before to how you treat me. If you choose to put me down or make fun of what I tell you, I will be hurt much more than I ever have before. And the more I love you, the harder this pain is to bear.

This is what so devastated Caesar when Brutus, next to his wife perhaps the most loved person in his quality world, attacked him. It was more than he could bear. He didn't fight back; he no longer wanted to live. It takes great care and consideration to be in love.

9

The Genetic Core of Our Personality: The Strength of Our Needs

The title of this book is *Getting Together and Staying Together,* but so far we have addressed only the problems associated with staying together. This is because most couples who are compatible and love each other enough to get married are almost always happy at the beginning of their marriage. It is when external control starts to take over that the marriage begins to fall apart.

But there is another problem of marriage, a problem that affects both the getting together before marriage and the staying together after marriage. This problem is so mysterious that few couples are aware of what it is. It is also such a serious problem that if even one of the partners knew about it before marriage, he or she might decide not to marry the other.

When we explained the basic needs, we stressed the fact

that these five needs are encoded in our genes. What we mentioned but did not fully explain is a problem that affects both marital and premarital relationships. This is the problem of genetic incompatibility. There is hardly a marriage that is not affected by genetic incompatibility in some way. But when it affects a marriage seriously, it can be disastrous unless the couple becomes aware of it and decides to work together to try to solve it.

It was because of just this problem that we heard from Ellen, the woman who was having an affair with Larry. She is the wife in a genetically incompatible marriage. Her e-mail follows.

Dear Dr. and Mrs. Glasser,

As Larry told you, I am the woman he has been seeing and with whom he shared the chapters you sent to him and Cheryl. I read them carefully, and then Larry and I talked them over, and he suggested that even though his marriage is really different from mine, I should write to you because you could be interested in how mine differs. In that talk, we decided to stop seeing each other. He was reluctant at first, but he agreed with me that if our marriages are to have any chance at all, we have to do this. Actually, I'm all for him trying to make a success of it with Cheryl. Having the affair has not been comfortable for me, and I want to concentrate on doing what I can to work things out better with my husband, Ian. I'm sorry to say this to you, but I was disappointed in the chapters you sent me. Not that what you suggest isn't good—from what

Larry tells me, it seems to be helping him and Cheryl—but getting rid of the deadly habits and reigniting sexual interest doesn't fit my situation at all. Ian and I don't use the habits on each other enough for them to be destructive; actually we are quite considerate of each other. Our problem, or I really should say *my* problem because Ian doesn't know I'm writing to you, is that I'm married to a man who has almost no interest in love. There's nothing to reignite.

You did mention that the strength of the needs follows a normal distribution. If this is correct, then Ian is several deviations below the norm in the strength of his need for love. As soon as I say this, I am sure you're wondering why I married him, and, of course, as soon as I read the chapter on the needs, I wondered about that, too. I have a very normal need for love, maybe even a little above normal. I married him because he is a very kind, if somewhat detached, man. He's also a very good provider. I don't have to work, and that gives me time to be the mother I want to be to our two boys. In many ways Ian is a good father. His parental love seems normal; it's his romantic love that's so deficient.

When we first got together, he seemed interested in sex. But I can see now it was all hormonal. At that time I had a lot of hormones too, and it worked for a while for me. We have two lovely boys to show for that effort. But as our marriage continued, and he sensed that I wanted more love than he was, I guess, able to give me, he dealt with my expectation by cooling off further. It was as if I was asking for more than he could provide. Also, when I say he cooled off, I don't want to intimate that he had far to go. At his best, he was never more than lukewarm. He's very uncomfortable with physical closeness. We even sleep in twin beds.

But please don't get me wrong. He's a good friend. And since we both like most sports, we go to a lot of games. He has season tickets to everything. Now that our boys are older, he takes them to weekend games. But it's not all sports. He'll go to adventure movies, and if there's a little love, he likes it. It's as if the character is doing it for him, if you can possibly understand what I mean. We also golf and ski, both of which I like, and while I'm not as good as he is I'm good enough. Besides, he's always supportive, and that helps.

Cheryl plays a lot of bridge without Larry, and Larry and I've gotten together weekends while Ian's at the games with the boys and she's at bridge. Like I said, I don't have to work, so now that the boys are busy teenagers, I started taking a class at the college, which is how I met Larry. We get together several times a week. I know it's no excuse, but it was my concern that there must be something wrong with me that led me to get involved with Larry. I hadn't had any sexual experience before I got married, and I wanted to see if I could have a normal, loving sexual relationship with a man. Larry assures me that there's nothing wrong with me in that department.

What I wonder is, am I mistaken? Am I missing something when I say Ian has no need for love? Could it be me? Do you think he would be more loving with another woman? I've talked to other women, and he's not the only man like that around. But from what they tell me he's more extreme than their husbands in the love department but much more friendly and supportive than theirs in other ways.

There's a very good thing that's happened with Larry. I've gotten rid of the headaches that have plagued me since I had my first child. I guess they started when I realized I was stuck in a no-love marriage. I was frustrated because if I hadn't been able to have children with Ian, I would have gotten a divorce. But now I don't want a divorce. I love my boys, and even Ian is happy about my getting rid of the headaches. I was pretty sure there was nothing wrong with me, that my headaches had something to do with my lack of love. So I went to the doctor and had a checkup, and I was right, tension headaches he called them. Can you blame me? I'm glad it wasn't worse.

Anyway, if you think you can help me, write me. You can write me at home. I take in all the mail, just put the letter in a plain envelope. Oh, I forgot. You can use my problem in any way you want in your book. I'm sure it's a fairly common one. Ian may be just a little more extreme than the usual "stay away from me" man. Do please answer so I know you've read this. Anything you can tell me that has a chance of helping us will be deeply appreciated.

Ellen

Ellen, with a normal or even above-normal need for love, found exactly the man she shouldn't have married. Given no other significant need-strength differences, a woman with a very low need for love might be happy with an easy-to-get-along-with man like Ian. Unfortunately, Ellen and Ian are not unusual; there are countless people whose need strengths give them personalities that make it difficult for them to be happy together. In theory, these people should never marry each other, but in practice they often do, and many stay together for years.

In this chapter, we will begin to explain that if the couple can become aware of this difference, knowing exactly where they are incompatible can help them if they decide to stay together. It also can help them if they want to try to work out the differences. There is no guarantee that they will succeed, but there is an absolute guarantee that if the couple doesn't know what these differences are, they will never work them out. With this in mind, we dropped a note to Ellen as she requested.

Dear Ellen,

We can see why what we wrote doesn't seem to address your problem as much as you would like. But at least our description of the needs helped you to understand what's wrong, and that's a start. We've been thinking about your problem, and although you can't change the strength of your needs, we don't believe the difference is so great that it can't be negotiated. Soon we will send you the rest of the book, which includes a chapter directly related to your problem but with the reference to your affair deleted. If this book gets published, we'll just use other names and other situations. Don't worry. We hope you will find the material helpful enough to share with Ian. If you do, we look forward to your feedback.

Cordially,
Bill and Carleen

The Genetic Basis of Our Personality

A lot of our personality can be attributed to behavioral role models like our parents, as in "He's a chip off the old block." But we also believe that a strong genetic factor could as easily make him a genetic chip off that same old block. It's really impossible to differentiate nature from nurture where our personality is concerned. Ian could have been adopted by very loving parents and still have turned out the way he has. As we will explain, all Ellen can do is try to teach him the value of loving. As yet, no one can change his genes, but helping him realize that his coolness may be genetic, that it's not his fault and she doesn't blame him for it, could be very helpful to both of them if they decide to try to work this out together.

Think of some people you have known for a long time. Many of them have a distinctive personality or way of approaching life that has led people to describe them with short, descriptive phrases. For example, Shawna is warm and fun loving; Jim is a macho, bodybuilding loner; Janet is a compulsive spender; Henry is a cautious saver; Carol is a risk taker; Harold is a playboy; Pauline is a very independent freethinker.

It is our contention that personalities such as these are strongly associated with a pattern, or *profile,* that can be created from rating the strength of the five basic needs. In this chapter, we use these need-strength profiles to compare the personalities of married couples like Ellen and Ian, as well as unmarried couples like Shawna and Jim.

Creating the Need-Strength Profile

To be able to compare a couple's profile, we will arrange the five needs in the following *order:* survival, love and belonging, power, freedom, and fun. Then, one at a time, we rate each of the five needs on a scale of 1 to 5, with *1 very low, 2 low, 3 average, 4 high,* and *5 very high* (see chart below).

Your Need Strength Profile

Fill in the circle above a number on the continuum to rate the strength of each of your needs as you perceive it to be:

	LOW		AVERAGE		HIGH
SURVIVAL	1	2	3	4	5
LOVE & BELONGING	1	2	3	4	5
POWER	1	2	3	4	5
FREEDOM	1	2	3	4	5
FUN	1	2	3	4	5

Record numbers from above here

Survival	Love & Belonging	Power	Freedom	Fun

Your profile is a five-digit number. For example, if all your needs were average in strength, your profile would be 33333. If all your needs were very strong, it would be 55555; or all very weak, 11111. But of course the need-strength profiles vary from need to need.

Keeping this in mind, let's take a look at how we would create need-strength profiles for warm, fun-loving Shawna and Jim, the macho, bodybuilding loner. Then we'll compare the profiles to see if they are compatible for marriage. Just from her brief description, it is obvious that Shawna has a strong need for love and belonging. Jim, a loner, has a weak need for love and belonging. Because she likes to be around people so much, her need for freedom is low. His need to be by himself working on his muscles indicates that his freedom need is high. Shawna has a low need for power; she wants to relate, not dominate. Jim, who builds big muscles to impress people, has a high need for power. Shawna's need for fun is high; it's a part of her described personality. It's hard to rate Jim's need for fun, so it's safe to call it average. Unlike cautious Henry, whose need for survival is high, or risk-taking Carol, whose need for survival is low, there is no indication from what we know that Shawna's need for survival is other than average. But Jim, as a bodybuilder, is likely concerned about his health, so he might be higher than Shawna in survival.

To use the order of the needs as stated above, Shawna's rating is: *survival 3, love and belonging 5, power 2, freedom 2,* and *fun 5:* a profile of 35225. Jim's rating is: *survival 4, love and belonging 2, power 4, freedom 5,* and *fun 3:* a profile of 42453. We rarely use 5 or 1 ratings unless there is an obvious indication of extremes as there is *in love and belonging and fun for Shawna* and *freedom for Jim.* In our experience, if there is a *two or more point difference between the man and the woman in any need,* that difference causes trouble. So if you compare their profiles, Shawna's 35225 with Jim's 42453, you can easily see that they have major difficulty getting along in four of their five needs, and even in survival there is a difference.

Suppose Jim and Shawna marry knowing nothing about the significant differences in their personality profiles. This happens all the time, because couples often have a great deal of sexual attraction in the beginning. Opposites do attract, because they both delude themselves into thinking, *With my love, the other will change*. But in a short time they have many problems. She would lack love and fun and be after him for affection, more social life, and more laughter. He would lack the freedom he wants, he would fight her effort to push him to socialize, and it's likely that because of his high power and freedom needs he would also ignore her request for more fun and affection.

But let's say they did marry and began to have the predicted trouble. Without knowing their profiles, this significant difference in four of their five needs is most likely impossible to work out. Their marriage would limp along miserably or end in divorce, and they would never know exactly what went wrong: that the trouble is more in their genes than in how they are actually treating each other.

Since there are countless marriages between people like Jim and Shawna, here is how we see these profiles working. Obviously, we recommend that all couples who are even thinking about getting married, while they are still infatuated with each other and open to communication, use this chapter and figure out their profiles individually, away from each other. The more honestly they do this, the better chance their marriage will have. After they are well enough acquainted with their own profiles so that they can explain them to another person, they should set aside a time when they will not be disturbed and share them with each other.

The first thing they should concentrate on are differences of two points or more, accepting that they exist and are not going to go away. The purpose of this initial discussion is to find out not only what the differences are but also to look at the places they are compatible. In Jim and Shawna's case, there really aren't any, but most couples have two or three compatible needs that can help them get along while they work on the incompatibilities. The good thing about the profiles is they show that it's not the whole relationship that's incompatible and, where there are differences, they usually can be addressed.

Before marriage is also the time to face any problems that have already surfaced in their relationship based on these differences. This will help couples to see clearly the potential for trouble if they do not accept and deal with the differences as early as possible. This is also the time to look for where they are already using the seven deadly habits and to start trying very hard to avoid using them. If couples who have significant incompatibilities don't do this early, preferably before marriage when they have strong positive feelings for each other, these differences may unleash a flood of deadly habits with all the misery that goes with them.

Ellen and Ian

Using what we have explained so far, let's now turn from the hypothetical Shawna and Jim to the real Ellen and Ian.

From what she said, the major difference in their profiles is in only one area, love. Ellen even said that Ian was relatively friendly as long as she didn't demand too much love, and that's a lot more hopeful than if he were both unloving *and* unfriendly. So let us construct a profile based on what little we know. Later, when Ellen reads this and, we hope, shares it with Ian, they can construct their actual profiles and more accurately pinpoint their differences.

Assuming that all we know is the difference in love, that otherwise they get along reasonably well, here are two possible profiles: Ellen, 34333, Ian, 31333. (Remember the order: survival, love, power, freedom, fun.) The difference in love is extreme, three points, and love compatibility is crucial if the marriage is to work. Bad as this looks, however, the situation is not hopeless. What we advise Ellen to do is to share all the material we will send her with Ian.

If Ian is interested, she should explain that she is not putting pressure on him for more love. All she is doing is showing him the extreme difference to see if he has any desire to try to do anything about it. With effort, we can always control our own behavior, even though our need strengths are fixed in our genes. Explain that the need difference doesn't make it impossible for him to love; it just makes it more difficult. Show him all their compatibilities and how worthwhile it is to try to improve this one area. Tell him she doesn't expect miracles, that if he starts by acting loving toward her, even if he doesn't really feel it, it's okay with her. She'll understand and appreciate his effort.

It is likely that Ian has some idea of his low need for love. This information will help because he'll realize it's not his fault and he needn't feel guilty. He'll also be able to see exactly what the problem is and that if he acts more loving it can help and can't do any harm. In essence, this is what all couples do with the need-strength profiles: pinpoint the problem and focus on what they can do to behave in more compatible ways. That's their choice. Jim and Shawna, with incompatibility in four needs, would have more serious problems than Ellen and Ian.

If You Are Single and Looking for Love

If you are single and looking for love, we suggest that you use what we have written here to construct your own profile. Then as you meet possible partners, try to evaluate how your profiles compare. You need not tell the other person what you are doing; just do it for yourself. It doesn't take much effort, and you can learn a lot about yourself and your prospective partner and get some idea of what your relationship would be like before you get to the point where you've moved in together.

You should look for compatibility in survival, especially money. In this area it is important that you be close. Big spenders have trouble married to ardent savers. Also look for freedom needs. People with a high need for freedom but who aren't aware of it get into marital difficulties early and don't know why. Marriage is about as unfree a situation as human beings have figured out to involve themselves in, and getting married does not change your need for freedom. In my experience, couples who love each other and who are aware of differences in their need for freedom can usually negotiate and work out this difference.

But by far the most important needs you should compare with a prospective partner are love and power. If you marry a high-power person (usually but not always the man), he can get very nasty if he's frustrated. Very high-power people always want to dominate and, often, to own their mates. They'd probably like to own everyone, but their mate is usually the only one available to them. If you don't want to be owned and bossed around, don't marry a high-power control freak. Ownership can lead to abuse, hatred, and even murder. The time to find out about this is before you marry.

The only thing that can counteract power is love, so check love for compatibility. Even two high-power people can get along if they love each other enough. One thing that will help two high-power people is working together toward a common goal. Then your power needs can help the relationship rather than harm it. There are many attractive high-power men around, so if you are a low-power woman you may be able to get along with one successfully if both of you have an above-average interest in love and if he uses his power to protect you. It takes real skill for a woman to do this, but at least if you are aware of it, you can try to accept his power as protective and see if it works for you.

Assuming you are a woman with at least average love and power needs, the one man you should avoid marrying—or if you've already married him, strongly consider leaving—is one with a *very low love need and a very high power need*. Assuming that all his other needs are average, this is a man with a 31533 profile. This is the minimal profile of a sociopath. Usually, he is more toward 21553, low in survival and high in freedom, but it is the X15XX profile to avoid at all costs. This man will pretend to love you but will exploit you and may even kill you. There are no redeeming features in the sociopath, and no woman can be happy or even safe with him.

The Marriage Prediction Experiment—Validating the Profiles

It was the surprising result of a 1988 experiment that led to my creation of the genetic profiles I have just described. For a long time, I'd had the idea that the strength of our needs had a lot to do with our personalities. It was also common knowledge that similar personalities increased marital success as I have just described. My problem was how to prove that this idea had some validity. As I kept thinking about it, I got the idea for the following experiment.

In a large meeting with about two hundred of my colleagues, we did the following experiment. To begin, I explained what I have just explained in this chapter, but in much less detail, and told them to break into groups of four or five. Then I asked each participant to write out the need-strength profiles of both his or her mother and father, rating each need as weak, average, or strong. (I used a three-step strength scale instead of the five-step scale I use now. But I don't believe that this small change made any significant difference in the outcome.)

Then on a separate piece of paper I asked each participant to rate the success of his or her parents' marriage on a three-point scale: 3 for a good marriage, 2 for an average marriage, and 1 for a poor or broken marriage. But they were to keep the success of their parents' marriage secret from the group.

Next I told them to show their mother-father profiles to the other members of the group. I gave them some more information on how the profiles could predict the success of the marriage. For example, if their parents had profiles like those of Jim and Shawna, I would predict a bad marriage.

Then I asked the other participants to look over each of the parent profiles and rate the marriages as *good, average,* or *poor* on the basis of these profiles. When all members of the group finished, they compared their estimates with the estimate that each son or daughter had kept secret. I then asked how many of the participants had rated the marriage accurately based on the profiles they had been given by the son or daughter of the couple they were rating.

The result was surprising. Just from seeing these need-strength profiles and knowing nothing else about the marriages, the results were far better than I anticipated. *Almost 95 percent of the participants were able to rate the marriages accurately based only on the profiles they saw.* This result validated the relative accuracy of the profiles estimated by the sons and daughters. We usually know other people better than they know themselves, yet the accuracy doesn't seem to drop if people rate themselves. What this experiment proved for me was that these profiles can serve as a powerful, predictive instrument for the success of a marriage.

I didn't do anything with this result until 1995, when I wrote the book *Staying Together*. Much of the information in this chapter was in that book.

Bill Glasser's Need-Strength Profile

To help you understand how to create your own need-strength profiles, I will use myself as an example.

Survival—3, Average

As I assess my life from the standpoint of this need, I am much more of a saver than a spender, but I like having the money to buy the few things that interest me. My definition of a rich person is someone who can buy any book (maybe thirty books a year) he or she wants to read, and by that standard I am rich. I am not a health fanatic, but I am careful about my health and I eat sensibly. I continue to have a strong interest in sex as I approach my seventy-fifth year, and that has something to do with at least an average need to survive. On the other hand, I know that I am not above average in needing to survive because I am not willing to settle for the status quo in any part of my life. In fact, all my life I have been eager to take risks and to explore new experiences and new ideas. Putting this together, I think I am well within the average range where survival is concerned.

Love and Belonging—4, Above Average

I am very much in need of personal love and intimacy, and I am also very concerned about the welfare of my fellow human beings. Most of my time is spent in an effort to create more satisfying schools for teachers and children. On the other hand, I have no need to socialize with strangers; I rarely talk or try to get acquainted with people who sit next to me on airplanes even though I fly continually. It is this reluctance to reach out to people I don't know, coupled with my strong need for closeness to those I love or know well, that make me think I am above average but not at the top in the strength of this need.

Power—4, Above Average

There is no doubt that I want very much to excel in my field and get recognition, or I wouldn't write books. But even in my field, although I crave recognition, I do not crave personal power. I don't like to give orders or tell people what to do for the sake of being in charge. I head a large organization, but I serve it far more than I run it, and I am always looking for ways to support the people who work there and to encourage them to develop new ideas. I delegate its operation to trusted associates; I listen to what they have to say and I almost always agree. But even if I disagree, I try to negotiate as long as things are at all negotiable. When they are not, as occasionally is the case, I go my own way. But when I do, I do not try to prevent those I disagree with from going their own ways too.

I make a very good living, and I want to be more than financially secure; I don't want to have to think about money at all. In a small way, I try to invest some of what I earn back into helping people use my ideas, and I never allow anyone who sponsors my presentations to lose money. I do not understand people who take from the needy or who lay off people when their company is reaping large profits, and I have no comprehension of people whose salaries are in the tens of millions. Even if they give to charity, how much better the lives of many people they employed could have been if they had taken less and used their skills to do more for those whose work has helped them achieve success.

In my relationships with women, I am not at all competitive. In my organization, women have an equal chance for whatever power is available and have availed themselves of this opportunity. I want to be recognized as one of the top people not only in my initial field, psychiatry, but also in education and management. To get there, I make an intense effort to persuade people to use my ideas, but I never try to pressure them to do so. I see myself as a leader, not a boss. This adds up to my being above average but not at the top where the strength of the power need is concerned.

Freedom—4, Above Average

More than anything else, this need is usually on my mind. I listen to people very carefully, but I can't stand it when people try to tell me how to live my life, or worse, try to make me do things I do not want to do. I think a major impetus for my success is the need to be able to choose almost all I do. For the unsuccessful, unfortunately, there is little freedom anywhere. I am a firm believer that people should not try to tell other people how to live their lives.

This book is dedicated to telling you what I believe will help you to deal with your marriage. But it is not dedicated to telling you specifically what to do with this knowledge: It is up to you to work this out for yourself. The most I do is make suggestions based on my knowledge and experience. This is the way I have lived my whole life, including reality therapy, the therapy I pioneered. Therapists are teachers, not preachers; clients are students, not followers. I am a strong believer in freedom of opportunity for all and the right to make choices.

At the same time, I believe in responsibility, and this belief is now stated as choice. People can argue about what responsibility is, but no one can honestly say that when we make a choice we are not responsible for what we choose. But I believe that we are not free to choose what we want at the expense of another human being or any other creature or the environment itself. If we don't all begin to take more responsibility for what we do to satisfy our needs, especially our need for power, we will soon become an endangered species ourselves.

Finally, it is difficult to reconcile my need for freedom and the restrictions of marriage. My late wife and I had many discussions about this, especially the conflict between my obligations to her and our family and my desire to pursue my career. We negotiated that difference almost all of our married life, and mostly we were successful, but the genetic difference here was extreme. We made a reasonably successful compromise, but to do this we had to talk and listen to each other, and it was never easy where freedom was concerned. I envy married people who have a lesser need for freedom; their lives seem so much easier.

Fun—5, Very Strong

Even more than freedom, I love fun. I like to laugh and joke. I strongly dislike seriousness if it is at all pretentious. I feel sorry for people who seem to have no sense of humor, but, for me, the humor has to make a point. Unless I can learn or teach from it, it is pointless. I don't have much patience for grossness or slapstick.

As explained, I firmly believe from personal experience that fun is the reward for learning, and I have been a passionate learner all my life. But I like to have the freedom to control my learning, so reading books has been my major source of fun since I was a child. For me, just settling down with a good book is an exciting experience.

If there is such a thing as mental health, to me it is most apparent in people who can enjoy laughing at themselves. An inability to do this signifies a low need for fun and a very high need for power. I would not advise anyone to marry a person with this personality. Power-driven people are filled with humor if they are making jokes at the expense of others, but they are not fun-loving; they are power-hungry put-downers, and I don't identify with them.

Fortunately, I am not so driven by power that I need power recreation. I like to play games and I like to win, but I do not have to win to enjoy myself. I get genuine pleasure when my opponent makes a good shot in tennis. And when the team I am rooting against makes a superb play, I enjoy it and clap. I said clap, not cheer—I'm not a saint! I like reading, travel, theater, art, music, and nonviolent movies, so I have no difficulty finding fun things to do. Based on this information, I think you have some idea of my personality and would agree with my need-strength profile of 34445.

As explained in the first paragraph of this book, after a reasonable period of mourning when my wife died in 1992, I decided I did not want to be lonely anymore. But easy as that decision was to make, it was hard to put into practice. I don't think it's easy at any age to find a satisfying long-term relationship. But at age sixty-eight, I was not prepared for how difficult it was to find someone new. As I thought about this, I began to think about what profile a woman would need to have to be compatible with my 34445. I was looking for someone who shared my zeal for teaching my ideas around the world.

As it turned out, I found Carleen, an instructor in my

organization, and we were married in 1995. Our relationship continues to be loving and strong and seems to get better and better as the years go by. But while we were going together, I was writing the original version of this book, so I asked her to help me by writing her need-strength profile. What follows is what she wrote. We did not show each other what we wrote until after we wrote it, and we did not change anything written here after we compared what we had written.

Carleen's Profile, Including What She Was Looking for in a Man

Based on what I know about myself, the following is a description of the pictures in my quality world of myself, my prospective mate, and our relationship. Most of these pictures have been in my quality world for many years; some are new pictures; and some are pictures I may have to remove as I continue to grow and evaluate their ability to satisfy my needs. But at the moment, what I have written is an accurate description.

Survival—3, Average

Since survival is connected with the drive to reproduce, and sex is part of that process, I believe my sex drive is normal to high. Mostly I think of myself as a sensual, exciting woman who enjoys lovemaking, especially if it includes exchanging lots of affection. I am fairly uninhibited and creatively expressive in my sexual play, and I expect the same from my partner. Although orgasm is very important to me, I consider it only one small part of the total sexual experience. I also prefer my lover to be slightly less driven by sexual urgency than I am. That way I feel safe because I am in more control of my experience.

Money is a necessary part of survival in our society, and I have enough to be relatively comfortable. I rarely worry about money. I don't waste it, and it always seems to be available when I need it. It is important to me to have an independent income. In addition to my full-time job, I have a small business and some investments to add to my retirement income for further security. I want a man who is also financially secure, not worried about his income, and willing to spend some of it having fun, preferably with me.

I am extremely healthy and not overly concerned about becoming ill. I am not an exercise fanatic and not particularly worried about my intake of fuel. I am not overweight, and I basically eat when I am hungry. I do not smoke, I do not drink alcohol excessively, and I avoid caffeine altogether.

I am neither a worrier nor overly concerned about change. I rather like new horizons and unusual experiences. I am spontaneous and able to pick up and go at a moment's notice. I am a risk taker to a degree. I am interested in a man who keeps himself physically fit and looks after his health. As much as possible, I want him to match my personality profile in the survival need, especially to be willing to take risks, too. Since none of this is extreme, I should have no difficulty finding a man who is compatible with my need to survive.

Love and Belonging—5, Very High

I come from a very affectionate family with lots of love and encouragement. I still crave being hugged and kissed, so I need a lot of affection from the man in my life. I like him to tell me often that he loves me, as well as everything he likes about me. I am convinced that lovemaking is a twenty-four-hour-a-day activity. It is expressed throughout the day by loving touches; warm, caring looks; little kindnesses; intimate conversations; and cuddling. I want a man who is present for me when he is with me. I like that presence to be time we just enjoy being together doing nothing in particular, our special time away from worldly distractions.

I enjoy being with people in almost every setting except at big parties or in very large crowds, unless they are an audience and I am the presenter. I would rather relate to people individually or in couples. In my work I deal with people, not things. When I find myself alone in my office doing paperwork for too long without human contact, I seek it. It is not that I mind being alone or that I fear it—I even enjoy some solitude every day—but I do not consider myself a loner. I really enjoy the company of a good friend or lover.

I have some very special women friends. I call them my "soul sisters" because we are of like minds. My daughter is one of them. I can talk with my "soul sisters" for hours, and we never tire of each other. I am looking for their counterpart in a man, someone who understands me and loves me just the way I am and who is of like mind. It is important that our philosophy of life be similar.

Because my love and belonging need rated my highest score, I keep a beautiful picture in my quality world of having a long-term, satisfying relationship wherein I feel completely loved and fulfilled. I can return the love freely, without inhibition and without fear of my love being rejected when the intensity is overwhelming. I will be sure it is right for me because when we are together I am happier than when we are apart. He knows how it feels to be in my skin and I know how it feels to be in his skin—we are that compatible!

What I also want from a man is complete intimacy. Nothing less will do for me. I am not looking to get married again, nor am I opposed to the idea, but whatever our ultimate status, I need a man who is willing to explore all the possibilities of a deeply intimate relationship with the creativity, honesty, and sense of humor it takes to keep love exciting, alive, and growing. He could expect no less a commitment from me.

Power—3, Average

Most of my power comes from how I feel about myself, not how much I need to control others. I have a positive self-image. I consider myself an attractive woman with the typical Mediterranean's dark, prominent eyes and sallow complexion. As far back as I can remember, I have attracted attention because of my somewhat striking appearance. I am fully aware that I dress to be noticed and use makeup with a dramatic flare. Even though I am over fifty, I look and act vibrant and energetic. I am an artist and enjoy using my talent to create the best look for me. I am successful because I am good at what I do and because I project a competent and beautiful self-image.

I have virtually no desire to control anyone else. Neither do I put anyone down in order to feel better about myself. I rarely compete for anything with anyone, even when playing a competitive game. I play for the fun of it, and if I lose (as I often do), I really win, because I enjoy the activity and the companionship.

I hate it when anyone makes fun of me seriously or in jest, and I especially dislike put-down humor of any kind.

Being taken for granted, or being ignored by a lover, is even worse. I want a man who is proud of my accomplishments and talents, not threatened by them, and who understands my lack of competitiveness and does not take advantage of it to get more power for himself. I do not want to be in a power struggle over anything with my mate.

Certain things are important to me and are tied to my self-image and power identity, and when I tell him what they are, I want him to respect them. Aesthetic experiences of all kinds are especially important to me. I am also interested in fashion and looking pretty in clothes, not as a symbol of power but for the aesthetic enjoyment of it.

My need for intrinsic power is high, but my need for external power is low. Put together, I think I am average in the strength of this need.

Freedom—4, Above Average

I believe we are all free. The only time we feel a lack of freedom is when we allow someone else to control us. My need for freedom right now is rather strong. In my life I have had varying degrees of freedom over the years, proportionate to the amount of control I perceived others to exert over me. Sometimes in the past, in order to get more freedom, I felt I had to go underground and live a secret life. Now I am living aboveground, and the freedom I give myself is matched by the freedom I recognize others to possess.

In my relationship with a man, I have no desire to restrict his freedom. What a foolish task for me to attempt, because it is impossible to accomplish! I do not demand exclusivity, for example, because demanding something I cannot control is an unrealistic expectation. He is going to do whatever is most need-satisfying for him anyway, no matter what I expect, and more so if I demand it. Therefore, I expect nothing but honesty. If he finds someone he prefers over me, so be it. If his preference is made known to me honestly, then he is gone and I am free to look elsewhere.

When I am completely in love with a man, I have no desire to be with another man, but I still feel free, because it is my choice to remain exclusive. I do not demand it of myself and do not want anyone else to demand it of me; it just happens. If I can fulfill all my needs with one man, why would I look for another? Perhaps for the thrill of conquest? But that is not getting me more freedom; that is getting me more power.

I feel exceedingly free because I am open-minded, accepting, and honest about myself. I want the same from my lover. I know that whenever I lock my mind in one position and refuse to budge on any issue, I become the one locked in while everyone else is merrily doing what they want to do no matter how much I suffer. I happily gave up that kind of thinking a long time ago. I am learning to let it go if it is out of my control. No one can restrict the freedom of my mind and choices I make but myself. Strap me in shackles and I will still find a way to be free!

Fun—4, Above Average

I need a man with a good sense of humor, who says funny things at the most unexpected times. I enjoy the spontaneous, the unpredictable, like a surprise letter, a winter vacation in the sun, sex in the middle of the night, Greek olives, the carousel ride at Santa Monica Pier, and a special man to share them with. I like to shop for bargains and have the sheer delight of finding the greatest one.

I laugh much more than I complain, and I want a man

who does the same. Some people have called me an incurable optimist because I tend to have a positive outlook and a joyfulness about me most of the time. I love learning new things, especially if I am good at doing them. I enjoy live theater, movies, art museums, traveling, and any creative project involving art and design. Even my work is fun for me most of the time.

I want a man who is fun to be with even when we are not doing anything special, someone who likes to listen to me and talks with me about anything and everything, someone I can laugh with and be silly with. At this stage in my life, I am ready to retire from my full-time job, continue to work occasionally at what I like, and have a good time being with a man who loves me joyfully and wants the same things in life as I do.

If we compare Carleen's 35344 profile with my profile 34445, you can see that these profiles are very compatible. With her I get a little more love and neither too little nor too much of survival, power, freedom, and fun. And our experience is that we are as compatible as I can imagine any couple can be.

In one respect, I see myself differently now after being married for almost five years to Carleen. The idea of being with anyone else is unthinkable, and there are other smaller changes, all for the better, that have moved into my quality world in the time we've been married.

If you are looking for a new love relationship or trying to improve the one you have, I again urge each of you to write your profiles out as we have and share them with each other. This will give fair warning to your prospective partner of what you are like and, if your partner does the same for you, fair warning of what he or she is like. If your profiles are not compatible, don't expect them to change very much.

No matter how well suited you seem to be when you start out, you and your partner still have your work cut out for you if either one or both of you fails to accept that your marriage takes precedence over what either of you wants. Where there are differences, find them early and negotiate. From the profiles, you know what differences to expect. Being surprised by an incompatibility is not good for your marriage. Most of these surprises quickly lead to external control and the seven habits. The whole point of the profiles is to prevent this from happening.

Profiles of Two Fictional Lovers, Robert and Francesca

Since their fictional lives have been made so public, I think it would be fun to compare the need-strength profiles of the lead characters in the bestselling novel *The Bridges of Madison County* to try to see what went wrong. Wrong, that is, if you are a romantic who was hoping for a happier ending. If you don't know the story or can't remember it, this is what happened.

Francesca was a forty-five-year-old, very attractive, starved-for-love housewife, living on a farm in Iowa with two teenage children and a good, if unromantic, husband, Richard. In some respects they were similar to Ellen and Ian, the couple we began this chapter with.

One day while Richard and the children were away for five days at the Illinois state fair, a tall, handsome, romantic, unmarried stranger pulled into Francesca's yard and asked directions to some interesting covered bridges that were unique to Madison County, the county in which the farm was located. He was a photographer who had an assignment to photograph the bridges for *National Geographic* magazine.

They were immediately and strongly attracted to each other, and in the four days until her husband and children returned, they were together day and night, making passionate love and leaving her farm only for the bridges, where she helped him photograph them. Then, because he was smart enough to know his limitations as a full-time lover and she was loyal enough to stay with her husband and family, they had to part. They never saw each other again. As ecstatic as their time together was, their parting was unbelievably sad. But if you knew their profiles, as I believe I do from the information in the book, you could have predicted that their love was doomed from the beginning.

I am relating this story to help you, if you are a woman, to understand how to figure out your profile and the profile of your mate. I am not saying that you should not have a passionate affair with a tall, handsome, romantic stranger if you ever get the opportunity. All I'm saying is that the better you know yourself and the man you are married to or living with, the better chance you have for a good relationship. This is the whole point of teaching you the profiles. The life you lead is up to you.

From what the author described, I would say that Robert, who was about fifty-five years old, was average in survival, love, and power (3, 3, 3), had a very high need for freedom (5), and a moderate need for fun (3), giving him a

33353 profile. I base this on the fact that he was divorced a long time ago, never remarried, and had no romantic attachments. He was a highly competent photographer and traveled the world by himself taking pictures. If he was passionate about anything, it was that the life he led gave him the chance to be free. He was a rolling stone who had not gathered any moss for many years. Since there was not much time to observe him in the short relationship, I am guessing that his need for fun was average.

Francesca had a high need for survival (5), a low need for power and freedom, both (2), or she would never have settled for so little, as she was educated and once taught school. She was a war bride whom Richard had met in Italy when he was young and romantic, but that had disappeared as he went back to the farm and brought her over to be his wife. She had never returned to see her family. She was a good mother and good wife, but the romance she had expected never panned out. She had a high need for love (5), and it was this that made her so reluctant to leave her children and a good, if unexciting, husband. But she yearned for romance and fell into the arms of Robert with a passion that astounded both of them. As with Robert, I am guessing that her need for fun was normal. Except for some initial flirting, their affair was mostly passion and misery. Her profile was 55223, compared to his 33353.

As much as Robert was able to love Francesca for four days, he was no Lochinvar. He rode off on his horse alone, even though none of her "kinsmen" would have been in hot pursuit if he had taken her with him. If she had pursued him, he would have been kind. But with his average love and high freedom needs, he did not have the long-term capacity to love her the way she would have wanted to be loved if she had made the sacrifice and gone with him. And he knew it. And she knew she could not go off with him. Her high survival need coupled with low power and low freedom needs prohibited such a spur-of-the-moment move. And her high need for love made it impossible for her to leave her children.

So she let him go, and he didn't protest. It was a sad but really not a tragic parting. I don't think they were nearly compatible enough to keep what was so wonderful for a week going for much longer than that. You can override your genes, but to do it for a long time takes a desire to negotiate that neither of them came close to having.

If you are interested in improving your ability to create your own need-strength profiles, try the following exercise. Pick a married couple you know very well. Then by yourself, or, better yet, with your partner, do what I did with Francesca and Robert: figure out their profiles. It doesn't matter if you make a mistake; neither this exercise nor your appraisal of your own need strengths depends on complete accuracy to be helpful.

When you have created each profile, see if these confirm what you believe is the success or failure of this couple's marriage. If the profiles confirm what you have observed, you have caught on to how to create them. Then use the profiles to pinpoint why their marriage is successful or unsuccessful. If you do this with a partner, discuss what the couple you profiled could do to improve their relationship.

10

The Only Person's Behavior We Can Control Is Our Own

Even though I explained in Chapter 5 when I talked to Cheryl that we can control only our own behavior, I'd like to show in more detail how this works in practice. Vera, unlike Cheryl, knew that her husband was unfaithful and came to me for counseling. I would like you to sit with me in my office as I counsel her. She was referred to me by her physician. All I knew about her when she came in was her name and that her doctor thought she would benefit from seeing a counselor. She was attractive, fashionable, beautifully made up, of average weight, and looked around forty years old. I took her address and phone number for my records, and then I started to work with her. I do not ask questions prior to the session because I don't want to bias my counseling by anything I say or do. What follows is not everything we said to each other on this visit, but it is the essence of our conversation.

"Vera, before we start, I'd like to ask your permission to tape what we talk about. I don't need the tape for myself. When the session's over, I'll give it to you. You can do what you want with it, listen to it or even destroy it. Is that okay?"

She nodded that it was fine with her.

Then I said, "Everyone who comes to see me has a story or something he or she wants to say. I wonder if you could tell me why you're here. We have plenty of time. I scheduled you as the last client of the day, so don't worry that you'll run out of time."

Her response was not unusual for this situation. "First of all, I don't want you to think I'm crazy. I have no idea why my doctor wants me to see you."

"I'll accept that you're not crazy. I haven't had a person I'd call crazy come to see me for two years. If I had to depend on crazy people, I'd have closed this office long ago."

"But you are a psychiatrist, aren't you? If you don't see crazy people, who do you see?"

"People like you. People like all the people you know. People with some sort of problem, or people who are sent to me because someone else thinks they have a problem. I guess you would fit into that category."

"Is having difficulty sleeping a mental problem? I went to my doctor for an annual checkup. You know, tests, X rays, the regular things. Then he asked me if everything was okay. I felt I had to say something, so I told him I was having a little trouble sleeping. The next thing I knew, he said I ought to see you. There's absolutely nothing wrong with me."

"Well, the last thing I want to do is tell you there's something wrong with you. I mean, did your doctor insist there was or tell you anything else? How well do you know him? It's very unusual for a doctor to refer a person for a little trouble sleeping."

"I know him very well. He's been our family doctor for over fifteen years. He's a caring man but not very communicative. When I asked him why I should see a counselor, he didn't explain it very well. He just said he thought it would be a good idea. He said, 'If you don't want to, you don't have to. It's just that for years you've never had anything wrong with you, and I remember that you always told me how well you slept. I don't want to give you medicine. You have good insurance, it won't cost you anything, just go and get it checked out.' So here I am. Check me out."

"Are you concerned about your sleeping?"

"Should I be?"

"Maybe, I don't know. It may be nothing. Are you married?"

"Why do you ask that?"

"Well, if you have a family doctor, maybe your husband talked to him and said something. If he did, he might have mentioned that he didn't want the doctor to tell you he was concerned. If you don't want to tell me you're married or if I'm totally off base for asking, say so. I'm not trying to make you into a mental patient. A lot of people who come to see me need to come only one time. But I guess I'm a little like you."

"What do you mean by that?"

"I mean you came here because you trust your doctor. And I feel the same way. I trust him, too. I'm glad you came."

"Suppose I have a problem. I'm not much of a believer

in psychiatry. How could you help me? You can't change the way my life is going."

"So you are married?

"Of course I'm married. Look, see the rings."

"I saw the rings. That doesn't always mean you're married."

"In my case it does. I've been married twice. I've had a lot of experience with marriage."

"Tell me about your marriage."

"Of course, that's it, isn't it? A forty-year-old woman has a problem, you think it's got to be her marriage. Okay, you're right, I do have marriage problems. Every woman I know has marriage problems. Half of them have gone to psychiatrists. They're all on Prozac or Zoloft or some other pill. But they still have marriage problems. Is that what you're going to do now that I've told you I have marriage problems, give me some Prozac?"

"No, I almost never prescribe medication. If you have a marriage problem, I'll offer to counsel you. If you want medication, you came to the wrong place."

"I asked my doctor, 'Why don't you give me some Prozac? That's what psychiatrists do. Why do I have to see one?'"

"What did he say?"

"He said what I told you. He doesn't talk much. I don't think they give him that much time to talk. He has a busy schedule. So when you counsel, what exactly do you do for a woman with a marriage problem? Tell her to stop depending on her husband? To get a life?"

"You're not coming across as a dependent woman. But you do seem a little angry. Could you tell me what you're angry about?"

"I guess I'm not doing too good a job of hiding it. I said to myself as I came up on the elevator, be calm, don't go in there and blow your stack."

"Your doctor noticed that, didn't he?"

"It's pretty hard not to notice, isn't it?"

"Have you ever told anyone the whole story?"

"It's not much of a story."

I nodded for her to tell me; I was listening.

"My husband is a big shot in the corporate world. If I mentioned the company, you'd recognize it. I worked for him as his assistant for ten years on his way up. We got involved. I got divorced and he got divorced. I wanted to keep working with him, but he didn't want that. The company didn't want it either. So now I stay home. I'm bored."

"You're very angry. I think it's more than boredom."

"It's a miserable déjà vu! It's his present assistant."

I looked at her, and she continued,

"No, it's not a divorce. He can't afford another divorce. He tells me he doesn't even want a divorce. He says he loves me, but he's weak, he can't keep it zipped. I don't have to be told the story, I know it all too well. If you can help me with my problem, I'd be impressed."

"Is he still seeing the woman?"

"He says he isn't. She's been given a new job where she can't see him at work. But what difference does it make? He's the way he is. It'll be someone else soon. I doubt if she's the only one."

"How does he treat you?"

"That's the point. The guy's a charmer. He doesn't know how to be anything else but charming. That's just the way he is."

"How did you find out?"

"I already knew the script. I saw all the signs immediately. I confronted him and he confessed. I think he wants me to know, just like he wanted his first wife to know. It's an ego thing with him. He's not going to change. He says he is, but he isn't. Do you think a guy like him will ever change?"

"You know him better than I do. Do you have children?"

"One, a daughter, she's twelve. If you think he's charming to women, you ought to see how he charms her."

"How have you been treating him?"

"Up and down. I don't know what else to do. One day I'm okay, the next day I'm on the warpath."

"What does he want you to do?"

"Forget it. Let it go. Accept him the way he is. Go buy some jewelry."

"What do you want to do?"

"Kill him one day, love him the next."

"In all the years you've known him, have you ever felt able to control him?"

"Control him? Doctor, where women are concerned, he can't even control himself. Ask him. He'll tell you that. He's been telling me that since I met him."

"Do you believe there was something wrong with what you did?"

"What do you mean by that?"

"Like it's your fault, that you didn't do enough, that you didn't love him enough. That if you'd been different, he wouldn't have done this to you."

"Of course I've had those feelings. How can I help but think that?"

"What good does it do you?"

"I can't help what I think, what I feel."

"Why can't you?"

"No one can. When you're upset, that's how you are."

"Who told you that?"

"No one told me that. It's what I feel, what I see everybody else doing. When people are upset they have no control over what they do."

"I don't think you can control your feelings. But I think you can control your thoughts. And you can control your actions, too. But maybe you don't want to control them. Maybe you're like your husband. He claims he can't control himself where women are concerned because he doesn't want to. Do you actually believe he can't?"

"It seems like he can't."

"Let's say he can't, that he's always going to be like he is. Is that the way you want to be? Do you want to be like him, or would you rather be more in control of yourself?"

"What do you mean?"

"I mean more in control of yourself in this situation with him. Not have all the ups and downs you've been choosing to have."

"What do you mean, choosing to have?"

"I mean just what I said. You choose loving him one day and wanting to kill him the next day. You choose the thoughts you're having and you choose the actions you take. How you feel and that you can't sleep aren't chosen, but they go along with the thoughts you choose."

"But I'm upset. I can't help myself. I told you that."

"I realize you're angry about what happened. And that it's possible your husband isn't going to change. Maybe this'll help. Tell me what you think about your marriage."

"I don't want to talk about my marriage. I don't even have a marriage."

"What do you want to talk about?"

"I just want things to be the way they were. I want all this not to have happened."

"Would you like to talk about the way things were? What was your marriage like before this happened?"

"Why do you keep harping on my marriage? I can't do anything about my marriage."

"That's not really true. You're the wife, you're half the marriage. Half is a lot more than none. You can choose to do a lot about your marriage if you want to."

"What could I do about my marriage? I've done everything I can. I don't think I can do any more."

"Oh, no. There're two things you could do right now, right here in my office. Two very big things."

For those who don't understand how I counsel, following choice theory, I believe that we choose all we do. My job is to persuade her that even in this situation, there are some choices she can make. Right now, she's choosing helplessness. It's not a bad choice, she could do worse. But the whole thrust of my counseling, which I call reality therapy, is for her to make choices that help her, choices that tell her, and maybe her husband too, that she is not helpless. She looked at me as if to say, what two choices do I have?

"Vera, you could choose to end your marriage or at least move out. Or you could choose to try to preserve it. My advice is to try to preserve it. You can always end it. That's always an option. You could talk it over with your daughter. She loves her father; how she sees the two of you is very important. She needs to feel as if no matter what you do, you're listening to her. She's twelve years old. At least she needs to have a chance to give some input into whatever is going to happen to her family."

"I don't have a marriage to preserve."

"I don't think your daughter would agree with that. But at least talk to her. If she wanted to live with him instead of you, she'd get a hearing. She may not want to lose her charming father. You have an unhappy marriage, Vera, but you have a marriage."

"You think I'm a lot stronger than I am."

"I know you're a lot stronger than you think you are right now. If you're looking for a counselor to feel sorry for a helpless woman, you haven't found one here."

"Okay, suppose I don't end my marriage. He doesn't want to end it. What do I do? What do I say?"

"What did you tell him when he ended his first marriage for you?"

"What are you talking about?"

"You must have talked. What did you talk about?"

"I told him I loved him. That he wasn't making a mistake. That I'd stand by him."

"He's made a lot of mistakes. But he doesn't want to leave you. Is that a mistake?"

"I don't know what you're driving at. Tell me what you're talking about."

"Tell him now what you told him then."

She looked at me as if I'd lost my mind, but I continued.

"If you have any love for him left at all, tell him you still love him. That you'll stand by him, and that he isn't making a mistake if he stays with you. How can this possibly hurt you? Put the ball in his court. It's his problem, not yours. Help him deal with it. You know how his wife acted when you came along. Do you want to act like she did? If he needs you now, be there. If he doesn't want you, let him tell you. Don't let him off as easily as she did."

"But I'd be giving in. That's what he wants me to do."

"Giving in to whom? Please tell me, to whom?"

"To him, I'd be giving in to him. My mother, my father, my sister, they'd all think I gave in. They'd have no respect for me."

"I'm going to tell you something that you don't expect me to say. It's something your mother, father, and sister would never tell you because they've never thought of it. And most of all, your husband's never thought of it either. It's a new way to think. It's like telling someone a thousand years ago that the earth is round."

She looked at me; I had her attention.

"Vera, if you do what I'm going to advise you to do, you're not giving in to him. You're giving in to your marriage. Half of your marriage is yours. If there is any benefit to what I'm advising you to do, you get half the benefit. If you give something to your marriage, you're saying to him that your marriage is more important than you being right. If you do this, you could ask him what he's prepared to do for your marriage. Not for you, but for your marriage. And for your child and his child; she's a part of both of you, she's a big part of your marriage. And a good part, you both love her. Don't you think he'll accept that no matter what he's done, he still thinks his marriage to you is more important than going off with her?"

"He's as much as said that several times, but I didn't think it was sincere."

"If it's not, you'll soon find out. But if you don't give him a chance you'll never know. Believe me, the woman he was seeing is more than happy to give him a chance if he asks her like he did you."

"But how do I do this? You pulled this out of me. I couldn't do this."

"You don't have to do anything. All you have to do is

ask him to listen to this tape with you. It pretty much speaks for itself."

That surprised her. She had forgotten about the tape. She hadn't really bad-mouthed him, there was no reason not to play it for him. She thought for a moment.

"I could do that, couldn't I? I could do it tonight."

"I don't see any reason to wait."

"Can I see you again?"

"You can see me, or you and he can see me. Or you can work things out on your own."

I put this counseling session in here to prepare you for the third part of choice theory, *total behavior,* which I explain in the next chapter. The first part is the basic needs, the second part is the quality world. And the fourth and final part is creativity, which I cover in Chapter 13. The more you know about this theory, the better chance you have for a happy marriage. In time you might want to read my book *Choice Theory,*[1] and then, *The Language of Choice Theory,*[2] which shows you how to put this theory to work at home, in school, and at work. And if you want to get a much better idea of what I did in this session, *Reality Therapy in Action*[3] presents many sessions like this one with Vera.

---

[1]New York: HarperCollinsPublishers, 1998.
[2]New York: HarperCollinsPublishers, 1999.
[3]New York: HarperCollinsPublishers, 2000.

11

Total Behavior

To begin, choice theory explains that all our behavior is what we call total behavior, an explanation that is much different from, and much more useful than, the standard explanation of behavior as a usual activity. When I say all behavior, I am talking about all conscious behavior that has a purpose. I am not talking about the tiny percentage of behaviors that are automatic, such as coughing or sneezing, or unconscious, such as dreaming. As I have already stated many times, all behavior is chosen. I'll explain that concept in more detail in this chapter.

As already explained, all our behavior is generated by the difference between what we want at the time, which is represented by a picture or pictures from our quality world, and what we have, which is what we perceive is going on in the real world. For example, most likely you are reading this book because you have a picture in your quality world of a better love relationship than you actually have right now. Driven by this difference between what you want and what you have, you hope this book will be a source of information you can use to get you closer to the relationship you want.

It is likely you are reading this book in the hopes of finding out what you can do to improve your love relationships, but this is not the only thing you could have done. You could have chosen to get drunk, a common choice for people who want quick relief from the pain of a bad relationship. You could have chosen to try to find someone else and become involved in an affair, or go so far as to leave your partner. You could have chosen one or more of the seven deadly habits and gone from there to arguing, fighting, or withdrawing, all very common choices.

Although you would not be aware that this is a choice, you could have chosen a physical pain, such as chronic headaches, or any one of the behaviors that are commonly called mental illness, such as depression, perhaps the most common of all the behavioral choices of unhappy people. The list of choices is endless. I mention only these few to show that, given the same unsatisfying situation, there are many total behaviors, mostly painful, we can and do choose in an attempt to make things better.

Choice theory, therefore, teaches something that most of you are aware of to some extent: When you are involved in an unsatisfying situation in your life, you cannot ignore it; you must do something. In many cases you are not even aware that what you are doing is a choice, as when you suffer from a headache for which the doctor can find no physical cause. But as I explain to some extent in this chapter and much more in my book *Choice Theory,* what you do that I call a total behavior is always a choice.

For example, many women come to me in my practice and say they are depressed. Even though a bad love relationship, usually marriage, is the most common source of depression in women, when I inquire about their marriage, often they tell me it is fine. But as we continue to talk about their marriage, it comes out that it is not nearly as good as they want it to be. In choice-theory terms, it is much less satisfying than the marriage picture in their quality world.

Later, as I explain choice theory and total behavior to them, they also find out that they are choosing to depress (the choice-theory terminology for depression). As they become acquainted with total behavior, they find out that if they are choosing to depress, they can make a better choice.

Even though all we do from birth to death is behave, as I explained in Chapter 5, it is obvious that behavior is much more than one thing. It certainly is action, or as I prefer to call the first of the four components of every total behavior, *acting*. But if it is chosen, it also must involve thinking, so *thinking* is the second component. Since when we are conscious we are always aware of feeling something, *feeling* is the third component of total behavior. Finally, our body is always doing something as long as we're alive, so what it is doing as we act, think, and feel is the fourth component of total behavior, *physiology*. Therefore, the four components of every total behavior are acting, thinking, feeling, and the physiology associated with them.

In the chapter with Cheryl where I explained the needs, I emphasized our feelings in an effort to show that when we satisfy one or more of the basic needs, the behaviors we use to satisfy them always feel good. Now you can see that I was talking about the feeling component of any need-satisfying total behavior. For example, if you hug and kiss someone you love, *the hugging and kissing is the activity.* While you are doing it, *you are thinking* about how much you enjoy doing this, and your thoughts may progress to a more intensely satisfying activity. All the while, you feel very good and may even feel better as the behavior intensifies. As all this is going on, your *heart and breathing* rates may increase and you may involuntarily moan with pleasure, which is the typical physiology associated with the total behavior called sexual activity.

As you think about hugging and kissing and about my claim that we choose all of our total behaviors, you may say that you are not choosing to moan, to increase the rate of your heart or breathing, or even to feel the way you feel. These are just happening as you hug and kiss. What you claim is true. All you are actually choosing is to hug and kiss and then to go on to choose sex. But could you experience the increased heart rate and the intense pleasure if you did not choose this activity and the accompanying thoughts? No, it would be impossible. In practice, we can rarely control or choose our feelings or our physiology, but we can *always* control or choose our conscious actions and thoughts.

Even though our control is not always effective, we are always in control of our own lives. Where marriage is concerned, this control is effective if we have a happy marriage and ineffective if we have an unhappy marriage. Therefore, to have a good marriage, we need to make competent choices. When I counseled Vera in the previous chapter, you could see that I did not focus on what she could not control, her feelings and physiology. I focused on what she could control, her actions and thoughts, even though, initially, she denied that this was possible. I did not attempt to help her to feel better, because choice theory teaches that without changing our actions and thoughts, it is impossible to feel better.

All we can change and, therefore, must change if we are dissatisfied with our behavior is how we are choosing to act and think. Since making a change in any component of a total behavior necessarily changes the whole behavior, it is correct to say that we choose our total behaviors. If we make better acting and thinking choices, we will feel better emotionally and have a more healthy physiology and, of course, a better marriage.

Even though it seems awkward at first, from now on I will use verbs to describe total behaviors because grammatically all behaviors are designated by verbs, never by nouns or adjectives. Therefore, we choose to depress (an infinitive) or we choose depressing (a gerund). We do not suffer from depression (a noun), and we are never depressed (an adjective). At first glance, this technical grammar may not seem very important, but if you incorporate it into your life, you will soon discover that it is. When you have a bad marriage and you think of yourself as depressed, or suffering from depression, you tend to feel helpless, as if this is happening to you from somewhere outside yourself, as Vera did when she blamed her husband for her helplessness.

If instead you say, *I am choosing to depress,* you are compelled to think of making an effort to find a better and more active choice than to sit around moping and hoping that someone or something will come along and make you feel better. You may begin to choose to think, *Maybe I ought to do something to help myself,* and then actually add some effective action to this thought. This is what Vera did when she decided she would play the tape for her husband. It is this effective voluntary effort that is the real message of this chapter.

What Is Misery and Why Do We Choose It?

Misery is the feeling component of a group of common total behaviors that most of us choose when we are in an unsatisfying relationship. The most common misery we choose is depressing, but we can also choose to withdraw, complain, go crazy, drink, or use drugs. We may choose to become anxious, tense, fearful, compulsive, or sick, a gamut of behaviors commonly chosen when we believe our marriage is not living up to its quality world picture. Usually preceding these behaviors, and sometimes accompanying them, is *angering,* as was seen for a while with Vera. Angering is the basic and most common of all the total behaviors we choose when things are not the way we want them to be. I think that anger is the only behavior that is encoded in our genes. We don't have to learn it; it's there at birth.

As difficult as it is for most of us to accept, we choose miserable total behaviors because we believe they are the best choices we can make at the time. The particular misery you choose is probably based on what you have discovered works best for you or what you have seen other miserable people choosing. I once counseled an eight-year-old girl who told me that when she grew up she was going to have migraine headaches just like her mother.

Finding out why you choose this or that misery is not particularly important. Choice theory teaches that what is important is figuring out how you can choose a more effective behavior, because until you do, your choice will be to suffer. Instead of expending time and energy trying to discover why you chose your particular misery, expend it on choosing a more effective total behavior that gets your needs satisfied.

Everyone who chooses to depress in a bad relationship wants to be treated better. Suppose you are a woman who is unable to get the love or attention you want from your husband. As much as you may want to, you cannot ignore what is going on. The underlying behavior that surfaces is anger, but if you choose to anger, in most cases you discover that angering makes things worse. It leads to fights, often to violence, and you, as the weaker party, usually lose.

But you cannot just stop angering. If you want to stop angering, you have to choose another behavior that, in effect, restrains it by replacing it. You have another behavior immediately available, which you learned when you were small: You choose to depress.

We all know from experience how to act, think, and feel when we choose to depress. Although you are usually not aware of it, your physiology is slowed down and you do not feel physically fit. Depressing is so familiar, so much a part of our common experience, that there is no synonym for it in the dictionary. You have been choosing it since childhood when you are frustrated, and you have done so for three reasons: (1) to restrain the angering that you know will make things worse; (2) as a cry to get help from your husband or from anyone else who might listen; and (3) as a way of avoiding doing something more effective, something that will take a lot of effort, for example, leaving your husband.

The first reason, restraining the angering, I have already

explained. The second is obvious; almost all of us are screaming for help when we choose to depress or feel helpless, as Vera did. Few of us choose suffering and then try to hide it. The third reason is less obvious and needs to be explained. For example, friends with whom you share your misery tell you, *Leave him*, and you agree. But in the same breath you say, *I will when I feel stronger*. Although choice theory teaches that depressing is a choice, it is not an easy choice, nor is it easy to make a better choice.

If you want to stop the misery you are choosing, you have to summon up the strength to make a better choice. It can be a relationship with a good, helping person such as a counselor who knows choice theory and who supports you and helps you find the strength to make a better choice, as I showed with Vera. But you can also learn this from a book. I have a lot of feedback from many people that they are able to do this from reading one of my books, and this book is no exception.

In my experience, most people have more strength than they realize, especially when they learn enough choice theory to know what's going on. They can use this strength to help themselves or use the encouragement of good friends and supportive family to solve the problem. What the knowledge of choice theory can offer is hope. It is the hopelessness of the thinking component of total behaviors like depressing that robs you of your strength and leads you to believe life is difficult and bleak.

If you are depressing, you are probably thinking that doing this is impossible. You may be saying you are not choosing to feel this way; it is happening to you. And you might add that no one in her right mind would choose to feel this way. What you do not realize is that you are no longer in your "right mind." As you continue to choose to depress, it feels as if your mind has lost its ability to direct you to help yourself the way you may have in the past. But it hasn't. Countless people overcome this feeling every day by changing what they are doing to a more effective behavior such as talking to someone who can help them see the alternatives.

You can now use your knowledge of total behavior to realize that you don't have to continue to choose to depress. You know that a better choice is available anytime you want to make it. In almost all instances, there are a wide variety of much more effective and, eventually, more satisfying, marriage-improving or marriage-dissolving behaviors than the painful and ineffective choice you've been making to depress.

Suggestions for Action

Take the time to say to yourself, and keep saying to yourself, "My marriage is unsatisfying and, for a long time, I have been choosing to depress (perhaps along with some other ineffective, miserable behaviors such as anxieting, angering, criticizing, complaining, withdrawing, and drinking), but now that I realize that I am choosing what I am doing, I am going to try to make a better choice."

It may take a while to come up with an idea for a better choice, but this book is filled with better choices, such as getting rid of the seven deadly habits. If you keep reminding yourself that you are choosing the painful total behavior you are feeling, you will begin to think harder about figuring out a more effective behavior. As you do, *these thoughts will give you hope,* and the self-chosen hopelessness that has dominated your marriage will lose its power.

As you gain a little control over the situation, you gain more hope. You begin to realize that what I have said is true: All the pain that you have been choosing has served no good, long-term purpose. You have kept your life together only by restraining your anger. You have made your cry for help, but you have stopped there. You may even have been able to excuse yourself for your lack of doing something better. But time continues to pass and you are really no better off where your marriage is concerned. So why continue to do this? Now that you have learned a little choice theory, why not try it? Let me suggest a specific choice-theory scenario that you might try. There is no guarantee it will work, but it certainly will not make your marriage any worse than it is now.

Let's assume that the vast majority of women who have locked themselves into unsatisfying marriages are not married to ogres. You do not live in fear of your life, and there are small islands of satisfaction in the sea of discontent. This point is important: What makes it bad is not so much the daily pain, it is that you have lost hope that it will ever be much better. But do you have to think this way? No. These thoughts are voluntary, and you can change them right now if you want to try.

To begin, wait for a time when you are alone with your partner and your relationship is neutral, that is, you are not arguing or fighting. Then, using a gentle, inquiring tone of voice, ask your partner the following question: "Right now are you satisfied with our marriage?" If he says "No" or "It's okay," as I assume he will, say either "I agree" or "It may be okay for you, but it's not enough for me." In the unlikely event that he says "Yes," say "Well, you may be satisfied, but I'm not."

If he asks what's wrong with the marriage or why you are so unhappy, or makes any reference to what in the marriage is not working, say "I don't want to talk about what's wrong because it doesn't make any difference whether we agree or disagree. Talking about what's wrong is not going to change anything. It's like talking about a flat tire; you can talk forever, but unless you fix it, it stays flat."

As he waits for what you are going to say next, add, "What I plan to do is try to get something going in this marriage as soon as possible that's better than what we have. If you want to work with me, fine. If you don't, I'm going to stop moping around and complaining about you, me, everybody, and everything and try to do something that we both enjoy. Life is too short to be unhappy, and I've been unhappy long enough."

At this point, if there is anything left of the marriage, he will wake up and begin to pay attention. He may ask, perhaps with some alarm, as he too is so used to the usual, stable misery that has become your marriage, "What are you going to do?" If he does, be prepared to ask with a smile that conveys the possibility that he too wants something better, "What would you like me to do? I'll do anything within reason you say, and I'm prepared to do it right now."

In the unlikely case that he suggests sex, be careful. For many men sex is the marriage cure-all. Your sex life is not insufficient because you don't desire sex or are incapable of enjoying it. It is suffering because you are not friends; most of the time one or both of you is inconsiderate of the other and you do almost nothing together that you both enjoy. This is the goal of what I am suggesting. If what I suggest is successful, sex will take care of itself.

After you pose the I'll-do-anything question, if he says nothing, or says he doesn't know what to suggest, be prepared to continue with no help from him. Don't be surprised if he draws a blank. If he were more aware and/or more creative, your marriage would already be in better shape. Expect this to happen and tell him that you are not depending on him.

Then give him a hug and a kiss and tell him, "Don't worry. I'll figure something out. But I'm sure that somewhere in your brain are some pictures of what we could do together that we would both enjoy." If you are completely stuck, say "Look, if you feel like it, we can talk again tomorrow. This is enough for me now. But keep what I said in mind. I'm tired of being unhappy and complaining about it all the time. I want to be happy and I plan to do something to find some happiness. I hope you'll help me figure out something we can do together, but if you won't, I'm still going ahead with my plan."

This is a big start, so don't push too far. You know enough about the basic needs to understand what he needs, too. You have worked out your need-strength profile and taken an educated guess at his. You have found that while you and he are not supercompatible, there is some compatibility. You have figured out what is in your quality world where marriage is concerned, and you have a good idea of what's in his, and it's probably not that much different. If he wants to talk further, which he may if you've stopped depressing, complaining, and criticizing, then your best chance is to ask him to read this book. If he will, you may be on your way to a more satisfying marriage.

At this point you've done about all you can. If he is still

not interested in working with you to improve your relationship, begin without him and then see what happens.

In any relationship, it is highly unlikely that if one person significantly changes how he or she behaves toward the other, the other's behavior will remain unchanged. The status quo is disturbed. There is hope. If you are the one setting in motion a positive effort to improve the relationship, the odds are that it will improve.

12

More Feedback

About a month after we sent Chapters 8 through 11 to Cheryl and Larry and also to Ellen, I got the following e-mail from Cheryl.

> Our marriage is definitely better. It isn't so much any particular thing you sent us, it's that when we have a problem, we now have quite a bit to talk about that we didn't have before. Instead of arguing or withdrawing, we now start looking for solutions. We even look forward to it, it's fun to use these ideas. But now that I think about it, there was something in the recent material, the idea that our marriage takes precedence over what either of us wants, that's now central to all our thinking. As soon as one of us starts in with anything, the other pipes up, "Is this good for our marriage?" It's no longer what I want or what he wants. I

guess you could say we look at what our marriage wants.

For example, I spend a lot of time playing bridge on weekends. I do this because I like bridge and Larry never seemed to care. I also did it because it ticked me off that he never wanted to come with me. It's not like he can't play bridge. He's a good player, maybe a little rusty on the bidding, but he can really play the cards. In the beginning of our marriage he used to come with me. But then I guess I got a little bossy and started criticizing his mistakes, and he stopped coming. The deadly habits killed one of the best things we had going for us in our marriage. They sure do rear their ugly heads at the bridge table.

But recently, out of a clear blue sky, he asked me, "Is that much bridge good for our marriage?" I didn't know what to say. He hadn't mentioned my being gone weekends playing bridge for years. I guess I'm a little addicted to it, but when he asked that question, I couldn't say it was good for our marriage. So I said, "You never seemed to care before. What's the big deal now?" He said, "It wasn't a problem when we weren't getting along, but now it is. I'm not going to make a federal case out of it, but since we've been looking at what's good for our marriage, that question seemed worth asking."

So I said, "Okay, if it bothers you, then let's negotiate. You brought it up, you go first. Tell me what you'll do that you think'll help solve the problem." That took him a little by surprise. Now he had to say what *he* was going to do about the problem, not put the burden on me the way he always did before. I felt pretty clever when I said that. But he said, "Cheryl, it's you who likes to play bridge. I'm not asking you to stop. I'm asking you to give me some idea of how you can keep playing so much bridge and help our marriage. I think that's fair."

If we're going to argue over who goes first, we may as well argue over my playing so much bridge. The way I see it, the whole point of negotiating is to solve problems, not to argue about them. So I just said, "I agree with you. I'll be glad to go first. How about if we plan something that we can do together on weekends instead of me playing bridge and you being on your own? Like I plan one weekend and you plan the next. Then, if you want to do something without me, I'll play bridge. I can always find a game."

Well, to my surprise, he said, "I like to play bridge. I'd play with you again if we could figure out a way to get rid of the deadly habits at the bridge table. I'm a little rusty, so you'll have to have patience with me, but I'd like to try." I said, "You'd really like to play bridge with me?" He nodded, so I suggested we start by playing on the Internet. I said, "A lot of people I know are playing that way. We don't even have to leave the house. Then we can play the same hand together and talk it over while we do it. You'll get practice and I'll have no reason to use the deadly habits. You'll be my helper, not my partner. There're games on the Net twenty-four hours a day."

So that's what we're doing. And it's working out great. He's a good player, and it makes the game so much more social. No one can hear what we say to each other. Now that he's had some practice, he's even been willing to come back to the club with me, and we're getting along fine as partners. If I hadn't written to you, this would never have happened. I mean, there's more, but I thought you'd enjoy this example.

The other stuff about the need-strength profiles was very interesting, but our profiles are fine. We did have a lot of fun figuring out some of the profiles in our family, especially our parents'. I think it's easier to figure out someone else's than your own. It was amazing. Just looking at those numbers painted such a clear picture of the marriages of so many of the couples we know. We both think that it was our genetic compatibility that preserved our marriage this long. If we'd been as incompatible as some of the people we rated, we wouldn't have made it this far. If there're any more chapters, send them, but we think we're in pretty good shape.

Thanks again,
Cheryl and Larry

Then, about two weeks later, we got a separate e-mail from Larry.

Dear Bill and Carleen,

I agree with what Cheryl wrote you. We are getting along much better than we have in years. And I guess you heard a while back from Ellen. I just wanted you to know that we've stopped seeing each other. I did talk to her after we got the recent material about the profiles, but all she said was it was interesting. She didn't want to talk with me about it.

The problem is that as much as Cheryl and I are getting along well, I miss Ellen. Or maybe I should say I miss having another woman in my life. The sex was important, but it's not just the sex. I guess it's the intimacy that I can't seem to get with Cheryl even though we're playing bridge and no longer arguing. If anyone had told me a year ago that this would happen, I'd have thought they'd lost their minds. I know this sounds strange, but it's hard for me to feel intimate with someone I'm so familiar with. She knows me too well. Maybe a part of intimacy is sharing your life, and I guess your body, with someone new. How do you get the old to be new?

I once read in a book that it's the getting together, the moving to closeness, the movement itself that's so exciting. Once you're married, that movement stops, or at least it slows down. I'm wrestling with the questions, "Is that excitement over for me? Will I have the strength to settle for just Cheryl?" But don't get me wrong, I'm only asking questions. I have no intention of giving Cheryl up now that we're getting along so well.

The truth is, I don't want a divorce. Like I told you the time I saw you, I like that Cheryl cares about me, and she's more caring now than ever. But I have to face another truth: I really don't think Cheryl's complaining was the real reason I did what I did. Even if we'd been getting along as well as we are now, I can't say I wouldn't have had affairs to get that new, exciting intimacy I seem to crave so much. I don't expect you to have the answer for the way I am or for what I should do. But who else can I ask? Maybe old age is the only solution, but I'm nowhere near senile. Could there be some kind of a pill for my problem?

Best,
Larry

Carleen and I talked about Larry's letter for a long time. His problem is neither unique nor exclusive to men. The only thing that's changed is that our society has reached such a level of affluence and free time that many more people are now struggling with the problem of excitement, a problem that historically was the prerogative of the rich and powerful. But in bygone days, the rich and powerful rarely divorced, and, like Cheryl and Larry, many of the people who are unfaithful today stay together. And, for that matter, people who are faithful separate. Infidelity is hardly the only reason for divorce. Larry will probably stay with Cheryl as long as she'll have him, and our guess is that even if she finds out he's unfaithful, she still may not want a divorce.

What we decided is that the real question Larry is asking is, "Isn't there a way to get more intimate with my wife than I have been able to get so far?" He admits that what we've suggested is helping, but it's not an answer to that question.

Dear Larry,

What you are feeling is a mystery of marriage for which we have no pat answer. You seem to be asking for a return to the feeling you had when you and Cheryl fell in love, to the time when you were still in the process of moving together. What you're asking us is, "Now that we're getting along so well, is our very familiarity preventing us, or at least me, from recapturing the feelings we once had?" Carleen and I have talked it over, and we don't think that you can recapture the feeling with Cheryl that you once had and that you crave with a new woman. Whether it's a car, a house, a new putter, the old can't compete with the new. Even Ellen couldn't compete with every new woman you may meet.

What you are asking for is impossible. It's like asking people to stop shopping and stop traveling. It would be like going to a movie and watching the scenery rather than the attractive people on the screen. In your request for an anti-straying remedy, you may be hinting that if we can't come up with an answer in some way it would be our fault if you don't remain faithful in your marriage. Like the prisoner said to the judge who sentenced him to ten years, "Your Honor, I can't do ten years." The judge said, "Then do the best you can."

So how well you will do the remaining years with Cheryl will depend on how hard you work on improving your marriage and how much both of you can accept that your marriage takes precedence over what you want as individuals. We don't think you're doing the best you can right now. Give yourself some more time.

Using what we've suggested in our book is a start toward where you want to go, but it is not a cure-all. It's up to you and to her to talk over your feelings and see if you want to try to get closer. You've rediscovered bridge. There are other things you can discover and rediscover. The more you attempt to involve yourselves in things you can do together, the better for your marriage and the less you will need what you crave. If you're asking us how to stop needing it at all, you're asking for the impossible. But what we will offer in the next chapter may help.

Best wishes,
Bill and Carleen

Then we heard from Ellen. Unlike Larry and Cheryl, she and Ian are not as compatible. But the fact that they have been able to deal with their major incompatibility may indicate they have more depth in their marriage than Cheryl and Larry. If they can use the need profiles to work out this problem, they may end up with a strong marriage. Ellen's letter follows.

The first thing I did with what you sent was read the part about the need-strength profiles twice. I think that what you suggested in your letter to me may be right. In the area of love it is not as bad as I feared: he is a 2 and I'd rate myself a 4. We could get along fine if he were even a 3, but that two-point difference is harder for me to live with than it should be. Although I had a lot of trepidation, I had to tell him what I'd figured out.

I told him about you and shared with him all the material you sent. He read it carefully and agreed with it. But as I feared, he said, "How can I be what I'm not?" And then he started to cry. In those tears, I clearly saw the whole problem of our marriage. I'd made up my mind that he was never going to be able to give me as much love as I want. In a sense I've been the storybook Beauty and he's been the storybook Beast. But in the story, Beauty learned to love the Beast the way he was, and that's what made the difference. Why can't I do that? It's not as if he has no feeling; he's not even as low as a 1 in love. He's a 2, there is some love in him. I'd just made up my mind that it wasn't enough for me.

When I realized that what I was asking of Ian was impossible for him to give I said, "Ian, please don't give up. Let's work out our complete profiles, not just the numbers for love and belonging." We did easily, and it turns out that we're not as compatible in the other areas as I'd hoped. He's a 32243. I'm a 34423. His need for freedom is definitely higher than mine. But when we compared his 32243 with my 34423 profile, it turns out that the difference in freedom is important.

Talking about those easily compared numbers has helped us to understand our situation a lot better than we ever have. I have a higher power need than he has, and I am naturally driven to try to force him to be the way I want him to be. As you pointed out, high-power people want to change the people they're with. He never tries to force me to do anything.

Low-power people like Ian have very little desire to force anyone to do anything. And when they are forced by someone else, they don't fight back, they do nothing. Also, he mistook my trying to get more love as me trying to control him and take away some of his cherished freedom. When we compared our profiles, it was obvious that with my higher need for power, I was coming across as begrudging him his freedom. I could see what was happening, and I immediately told him I didn't begrudge him anything. He could have all the freedom he wanted. He isn't a 5, he's a 4. It's no big deal. I think 5's are freedom fanatics and get crazy when anyone even breathes in the direction of taking some of their freedom away, but that's not Ian.

He was worried that I'd mind if he preferred to take the boys to baseball games instead of me. I don't mind at all. If he doesn't have to protect his need for freedom, I think he'll be perfectly willing to be closer to me, and that's what seems to be working. I don't mean all hugs and kisses, but compared to how he's been, a lot closer.

I have to tell you that running those complete profiles made it crystal clear. I also have to tell you that I still want more love than he's comfortable with. And from the profiles, he says he can understand why I want more love, and he doesn't at all resent me wanting it just as I don't resent him for wanting more freedom. We talked honestly about my above-average need for love and his above-average need for freedom. He believes there's a big difference between freedom and love. All I have to do to give him his freedom is to leave him alone. But for him to be more loving, he has to be active, to do things that he really doesn't feel like doing. I began to see his point and told him to relax and talk to me more about it.

He said that even though I rarely come right out and criticize him, he couldn't help mistaking my dissatisfaction with his passivity about love as criticism, which is external control, isn't it? And that made him afraid to try to make any effort to love me. He was concerned he'd do a lousy job and get more criticism from me. What this showed both of us is how destructive criticism is. As soon as he felt he was incapable of loving me the way I wanted to be loved, he turned my felt criticism into self-criticism. He was not only resentful of me, he pulled away from me. He thought I was attempting to rob him of his freedom.

But now it's all out on the table. He accepts that I need more love than he gave me. I appreciate any effort he makes to get closer to me and don't ask for more. The way it's worked out, the more we accept that we're different, but not so different that we're totally incompatible, the closer we get. If we hadn't focused so much on our love differences and instead figured out our whole profiles, it would have saved a lot of misunderstanding. The getting closer is slow, but it's steady, and we feel better and better about our marriage.

The way we see it, a married couple doesn't have to be compatible in every need to make a success of their marriage. It just takes a willingness to talk about it without putting each other down and for each one to give a little. If they will accept each other where they are incompatible and make an effort to be understanding of each other's needs, most differences can be worked out.

Best regards,
Ellen and Ian

13

Creativity, the Final Component of Choice Theory

As we discussed in Chapter 3, when tension arises in relationships other than marriage, usually you can just walk away for a while, and you're both relieved. When the tension lifts, you can get back together. You are not tied to each other. When you get back together, the problem may have been solved by time. But in marriage you are tied to each other, and walking away is not an option unless you are willing to jeopardize your marriage.

It is because you can't walk away that the seven habits take a bigger toll on marriage than on any other relationship. Each partner wants to have the last word, to argue to the bitter end, to keep trying to change the other, to get the other to admit wrong, to blame the other for the problem, for not being sensitive to "my needs," and for not trying "to work things out."

How to relate to each other without doing this is the

ultimate challenge of the marital relationship, and everything we have suggested so far in this book are ways to avoid this situation. What we have explained is tangible and, from personal experience, we know it works. But there is some further information that we would like to share with you about creativity. It is so intangible that it's difficult to explain, but we will do our best to help you begin to use it in your marriage, especially when nothing else seems to help. It is most helpful when you are in a conflict, the most difficult of all relationship problems and especially common to the bound-together relationship that is marriage.

Conflict

Conflict occurs when you have two contradictory pictures in your quality world and there is no way to reconcile them. In a marriage like Ellen's, for example, you may want to leave because you are not getting nearly enough love and attention, but you do not want to break up the family. Your husband is a good provider and a good father, but you are starved for love. In this situation, there is no behavior that will work—you can't both leave and stay—and no one can help you. When you are in a conflict, no matter what you choose to do, if you cannot reconcile the contradictory pictures, the conflict remains. Except for restraining the angering, all the suffering you are choosing—for example, your choice to depress—is in vain. But when you are in a conflict, there is another option you can rely on, your creativity.

The Choice-Theory Explanation of Creativity

In Larry's case, and Cheryl's too—in fact, with all dissatisfied couples—the best way to add more closeness to their marriage is to be creative. And the good news is that creativity is available to all of us; what we lack is how to access it. We have in our brains what I call a *creative system*. This system is always paying attention to what we are trying to do with our lives, even though we are rarely aware of the system itself. We believe that if we are aware that such a system exists in our brains, we can use this awareness to help us access it.

We become aware of its power when it offers us a novel idea or a new insight as it offered Edison with the electric light and Einstein with the theory of relativity. But creativity is not restricted to genius. Everything in the world that is not natural is the product of human creativity; things as mundane as the Post-it note are valuable but hardly the work of genius.

Like all behaviors, a new or creative behavior is a total behavior, but the creativity need not be in any more than one component. It may be a new activity, a new idea, a new feeling, a new physiology, or any combination. How all this happens is beyond the scope of this book (see Chapter 7 of *Choice Theory* for details), but here I'd like to explain how it can work in marriage by offering new ways to solve problems.

An unloved married woman's creativity may tell her, *Get out, don't worry about the future, just leave and take a chance that you will be able to cope without him.* This may not seem that creative, but for her it is. It's so new and so drastic, so impulsive and so far-fetched, that she may not seriously consider it. But this is how your creative system works. It does not necessarily come up with anything sensible or even moral, or even something that new. Certainly leaving a husband is hardly a new idea. All it has to be is *new to her.* If it fulfills this criterion, it is creative.

If the creativity is in the form of a new idea or a new thought, it is usually only offered. It is up to her to take it or leave it. But sometimes it goes beyond offering and actually invades your thinking with a delusion or invades your perceptions with a hallucination. How to deal with this is covered in the books *Choice Theory* and *Reality Therapy in Action.* If your creativity offers you an idea or a behavior that you are able to recognize as new, you don't have to act on it any more than you have to act on what is offered to you in dreams. Dreaming is pure creativity.

In this instance, if she gets the idea to get up and leave, she can take action on it if she wants to. What she actually chooses may not be the smartest thing to do, but that's up to her to decide, especially if what is offered is destructive or self-destructive, as when it may offer murder or suicide. But please be clear that if it offers her the idea to kill her husband and she carries it out, she is still responsible. Our legal system sometimes allows people to escape responsibility for what they do by blaming their creative system for what it offered, as in temporary insanity. But that is not the fault of the legal system. It may be the fault of psychiatry for confusing creativity with mental illness.

When we are in a conflict, the usual, and extremely uncreative way, to deal with it is to choose to depress or withdraw. When we choose these common forms of misery, it feels as if we're stuck in the feeling itself. Doing something new in this situation is the last thing we think about.

But creativity has been built into our brains as a way to get ourselves unstuck, a way to get going when all you can think of is, "It's hopeless." Your creative system is never stuck. It's always working to come up with something to do, but you have to listen to it, give it a real hearing. If life offers you a bag of lemons, don't throw them away, make lemonade.

When Martha found herself in a sexless marriage, she got the creative idea (again, for her, not for anyone else) of showing her husband some videos. Many women would have dismissed this idea as ridiculous, but she followed through. What is important is to accept the fact that we are continually and amazingly creative, but most of us never tap into this potential because it's hard to accept much of our own creativity. When we are in a difficult situation such as an unhappy marriage, we certainly don't feel creative. We stick to a set of habitual, uncreative behaviors, as Larry did in looking for other women. With them he may have been creative, but if he wants to be happy with Cheryl, he needs to tap into his creativity for new ways to connect with her.

The best, if not the only, way to add more closeness to a long-term relationship is to be creative, to continually look for new things to do with each other in the marriage. To get the system working for you, the best thing to do, by yourself or, better still, together, is to be on the lookout for what each of your creative systems offers that is new and may, if put into practice, bring you closer. To make yourself more accessible to it, make up your minds that you don't want the same old thing, you want variety. Then wait.

In the case of Carleen and me, this book is a creative product of deciding to do something together that has a purpose. We want to make a difference, a contribution to better understanding the marriage relationship by shedding light on some of its mysteries. It's up to you to judge whether what we did is creative, but we know that writing it together has helped us see each other with renewed depth and has added a lot to our closeness as a couple.

If you open yourself up to your creative system, be prepared to be offered any number of stupid or worthless thoughts. Just because you reject them, don't criticize yourself or each other no matter what comes to mind. Self-criticism especially turns this system off. Be patient. Don't use the seven deadly habits on yourself, and your creative system will produce. Every idea in this book that helps your relationship will give you more access to your creative system. If you use the ideas, you will have an opportunity to create the closeness your marriage needs to endure.

There is no way you can spend a lifetime happily with another person without a lot of creativity. It's not so much a matter of turning it on, it's already on. It's much more a matter of not turning it off. We wish we could explain creativity in a more specific, more accessible way. But, unfortunately, this is all we can do. The rest is up to you. Creativity is a mystery that goes far beyond marriage. Mysterious as it is, creativity is a fundamental property of all life.

14

A Happy, Creative Marriage

When I was writing the first edition of this book in 1994, I asked in my *Institute Newsletter* for members to send in anything they do that has made their marriages happy. I expected to get a lot of answers, but the responses were few and very sparse. I have wondered about this a great deal. Are there so few happy marriages? This may be the case, but I think the answer is something else. I think that what makes a marriage happy is, for most satisfied couples, so ordinary that few thought they had significant ideas to contribute.

The couples who wrote stressed the importance of friendship and made an effort to remain good friends. They don't let misunderstandings take root and become problems; they talk and listen to each other even when they are upset. Some, but not all, mentioned sex. Those who did said they continued to be willing learners and listeners and tried to be creative in bed, but it was the friendship that kept the sex good. These couples confirm a major message of this book: Treat your spouse as you do your best friend.

One of the few extensive responses came from a couple who have been happily married for more than twenty-six years. The response was so appropriate and well written that I would like to close this book by sharing it:

1. We have had at least five different relationships with each other over the past twenty-six years.
2. Celebrate the presence of each other many times each day: excited greetings, enthusiasm on the phone, frequent "I love yous," singing songs about each other.
3. Always create dates with each other even during the child-rearing years and the busiest of times.
4. Nurture each other. Look for ways to support each other physically and emotionally; for example, make favorite meals, drive each other to work during storms, consult about business, give massages when watching TV.
5. Take the risk of telling each other what you want and also risk telling each other what you see as not right.
6. Love each other unconditionally. Don't hold out expectations that either raise or lower the amount of love. Love must be freely given.
7. Give freedom to be his or her own person. Accept differences. Honor the boundaries between who one is and who the other is.
8. Look to each other as best friends. Day after day, think and act together as best buddies.
9. Know how to laugh, be silly, and have fun together, with no concern about being embarrassed; for exam-

ple, speaking in made-up foreign languages, humming and squeezing each other to make songs.

10. Keep sex lively and always growing in mutually agreed-upon experimentation.
11. Enjoy making lists together.

We are impressed with how much thought and effort this couple has put into their happy marriage. This does not mean that it has all been rosy; there are no totally rosy marriages. But this couple, without reading this book, confirms most of what we have written. What interests us most about their list is the first point, their claim to have had at least five different relationships in the last twenty six years. I wondered what these were and asked for more detail.

Here is their description of the various roles that each has played in the marriage.

- She is a young, bright, serious, protected, inexperienced college student.

  He is a young, creative, rebellious, lively high school teacher.

- She is an earth mother, bearing a child, a wonderful cook, weaver, and craftsman.

  He is an alternative-culture community activist, creating new forms and systems in schools and neighborhoods.

- She is an entry-level career woman, provider of family income, leader in her organization and community.

  He is out of institutionalized work life, gives primary care to their child; a poet, thinker, into meditation.

• She is an experienced executive, a national leader in her profession, with a fairly high income; a role model to their teenager daughter.	He is an entrepreneur, co-owner of a construction company, active in church leadership, staff development in social service agency.
• She is an executive, developing body awareness, foreign language, and new spiritual dimensions, with a deep appreciation for her husband.	He is a business consultant, pioneering new methodologies for organizations to operate effectively, with a deep appreciation for his wife.

Both were aware of the need for new life roles in any long and necessarily changing relationship and were willing to make the effort to create these roles. What they did is so much more satisfying than doing the same things with a variety of mates through affairs and multiple marriages.

Now, five years later, we asked this same couple to give us an update. This is what they wrote:

> Wanting to grow closer, stay monogamous, and be abundantly alive in middle age, about four years ago we began exploring new ways of being intimate. The breakthrough discovery we made together was finding the ancient system of tantra kriya yoga. Having experienced and practiced the techniques for three years, we now are able to love one another without conditions or bartering. There is an unwavering trust at the core of our relationship. Enjoying ecstatic sex on a continual basis spreads to all aspects of our lives. As certified

teachers, we share the tantra yoga system with hundreds of others in the central part of the United States through workshops we lead. The key is being fully aware that we are a creative couple without limits.

Will You Help?

If you have been helped by this book, we would like to find out what it was that helped you. The only way that we can get this information is if you write and tell us. We may not be able to answer your individual letters if we get a lot of them, but we will put together a composite answer that we are sure will be both interesting and useful and mail it to all who write. Write to us at:

William Glasser, M.D., Inc.
22024 Lassen St., Suite 118
Chatsworth, CA 91311
E-mail: wginst@earthlink.net